BODY

The Essentials of Health & Wellness

D1051958

Ryan Carnahan, RMT, DCH

Book One

Library and Archives Canada Cataloguing in Publication

Carnahan, Ryan, 1973-
Body: the essentials of health and wellness / Ryan Carnahan.

Includes bibliographical references.
ISBN 978-0-9811246-1-2
1. Self-care, Health. 2. Well-being. I. Title.

RA776.95.C37 2009   613   C2009-904197-9

Illustrations by Alisha Reilly-Roe
Editing by Linda Parsons
Book design by Linda Parke

First Printing January 2010

Ryan Carnahan
Vancouver BC Canada
www.ryancarnahan.com

To my mom and dad.
Thank you for always being there.

NOTE TO THE READER

The information, ideas, and suggestions in this book are not intended to be a substitute for consulting with your physician and obtaining medical advice and supervision regarding any activity, procedure, or suggestion that might affect your health.

It is important to assume responsibility for your own actions with regard to your health, wellbeing, and safety.

Neither the author, nor the publisher shall be liable or responsible for any loss, injury, or damage allegedly arising as a consequence of your use or application of any information or suggestions in this book.

Any website addresses or links contained in this book may have changed since publication and may no longer be valid.

ACKNOWLEDGEMENTS

I would like to thank those individuals who have influenced, inspired, and shaped the foundations for this book. Without these people, this book would not exist. I feel fortunate to have these people in my life and the gifts they have given me.

I thank my father George Carnahan for guiding me toward a fulfilling career in natural health care, and my mother Vivian Carnahan for the love and support she has given me throughout my life.

Deepest gratitude to those teachers who have guided me on this path of life and whose influence can be felt in this book: Sensei Chris Taneda for teaching me how to move my body and focus my mind; Murray Feldman for introducing me to the world of homeopathy; Dr. Jonn Matsen for 13 years of learning by osmosis in his clinic; and Geoff Gluckman for teaching me about movement, posture, and self-responsibility. Thank you all for everything that you have shared with me so that I may share with others.

Other people who have specifically been a part of this book that I would like to thank: Jill Carnahan for her review and feedback of this book; my editor Linda Parsons for her keen eye, insight, and commitment—you helped bring the essence of this book to the forefront—thank you.

Warm thanks to my good friend and artist Alisha Reilly-Roe, whose artwork added a whole new dimension to this book that words alone could not do—thank you.

To Dr. Jason Loken, for your friendship, support, and kinship—your insights helped take this book to a whole new level. Thank you.

And finally to my loving wife Kira—thank you so much for your patience, input, and support while writing this book—I could not have done it without you. Your professional insights as a naturopathic doctor, your deep wisdom, and the light in your eyes have all guided me on this journey. Thank you so much.

CONTENTS

CHAPTER 2: FOOD   25

INTRODUCTION

"What can I do to help myself?"

People have been asking me this question on a near daily basis for over 15 years. Practitioners in the healing arts are faced with a dual challenge—to help people heal and to educate and empower people to heal themselves. Most often the latter gets overshadowed by the limitations of practice because time constraints prevent lengthy discussions on self-help solutions. This book was written to fill the need of those seeking the answer to this question.

With such an overwhelming volume of health information available today, it's easy to get confused. To demystify the process and eliminate complexity, I have provided a simple, easy to understand foundation from which everyone can start their self-educating, self-empowering, and self-healing journey.

Advancements in technology, innovative treatments, new supplements, and medications will continue to emerge but the fundamental, essential requirements for good health and wellness will always remain the same.

In this first of three books, you will be introduced to the essentials of health and wellness relating to the "Body". In Books 2 and 3 you will learn about the other two equally important aspects of health—"Mind" and "Spirit".

The books are meant to be read in order. Take your time with each chapter and revisit the information often if needed. Remember, although the content in this book is interesting—it can only be beneficial when *applied*.

It is my sincere hope that you find the information contained within these chapters useful and indeed applicable.

The power to heal yourself is inherent within you and begins in the most fundamental form as knowledge. With knowledge comes choice. That choice belongs to you.

In answer to your initial question of what you can do, I offer you this book. This is what you can do.

To your health and wellness,

Ryan

Chapter (1)

MOVEMENT

Movement is one of the most essential components to all life—your body cannot survive without it. Every living tissue requires movement to flourish, from your muscles and joints to your organs and cells.

EXERCISE AS MOVEMENT

Exercise makes you stronger, improves your cardiovascular system, and is essential for maintaining a healthy weight. But exercise also has many other lesser known benefits.

Did you know that exercise is capable of enhancing your immune system, calming your nervous system, improving your sleep, balancing your hormones, and stimulating your digestion? Did you know that exercise can improve mental functioning and enhance learning and memory?[1]

Exercise can even reduce the incidence of cancer, heart disease, diabetes, osteoporosis, and other chronic diseases.[2,3] It can relieve depression, improve energy levels, promote mental and emotional well-being, and stimulate your body's detoxification system.[4,5]

Every cell in every system of your body derives benefit from exercise.

> *Every cell in every system of your body benefits from exercise.*

USE IT OR LOSE IT

When applied to physiology, the "use it or lose it" principle means if you do not use a function in your body you will eventually lose the ability to perform that function. For example, if you never raised your arms over your head for many years, you would eventually lose the ability to do it with the same balance, strength, flexibility, endurance, and coordination that you have now.

Try it now. Lift your arms up to your ears keeping your arms straight and your palms facing inwards. Can you do it easily? Do your shoulders feel tight or loose? How about the rest of your body? Can you comfortably sit cross-legged on the floor or touch your toes easily? Turn your head left and right—does your chin reach your shoulders?

If your body feels flexible and strong, then your lifestyle probably includes some form of regular movement. If it feels stiff or rickety, then it may be time for a tune-up. That tune-up can start right here and now with the **first body essential to health and wellness—*movement*.**

THE SEDENTARY LIFESTYLE

Living a *sedentary lifestyle* with little physical movement contributes to a decreased capacity of various bodily systems, especially the musculoskeletal system.

The sedentary lifestyle has become the norm of modern day society for most North Americans. It could also be called the "not using it and losing it" lifestyle. Failing to move your body properly on a daily basis can prevent you from experiencing vibrant and abundant health.

SEDENTARY DEBT

Sedentary debt is the number of hours you spend lying or sitting down in the course of your average day. Each day the number of hours spent being sedentary is tallied up as a debt in *movement*. Like a credit card or any other type of debt, this sedentary debt can both accumulate and be repaid.

YOUR HEALTH ACCOUNT

Your *health account* is your body's bank account that keeps track of your *health dollars*. Health dollars are credits that contribute to your vitality, longevity, enjoyment of life, sense of peace, and physical function.

Health dollars are earned and spent by physical, mental, emotional, and spiritual actions and intentions. As long as you maintain a positive balance in your health account with an abundance of health dollars, you reap the rewards of increased vitality, longevity, and vibrant aliveness.

Conversely, when your health account becomes depleted, *health bankruptcy* occurs resulting in a variety of health problems—aches and pains, lack of energy, and a general feeling of *dis*-ease.

What kind of investment are you making? Are you devoting the same level of care with your health as you are with your money? Investing wisely in your health and well-being will yield high returns.

SEDENTARY DEBT AND YOUR HEALTH ACCOUNT

The bottom line is sedentary debt *subtracts* health dollars from your health account, robs you of your well-being, vitality, longevity, and physical function—and worse can result in health bankruptcy.

But the good news is like other debts, sedentary debt *can* be paid off. Not only can it be paid off, but health dollars can be added to your health account to create a positive balance.

You will learn exactly how to do this later in the chapter, but first take an inventory of the amount of sedentary debt you accumulate in a day.

CALCULATE YOUR SEDENTARY DEBT

Write down the number of hours (to the half hour) per day you spend either lying or sitting down in each of the following:

Lying in bed (including sleep)   _____

Sitting in transit   _____

Sitting at work   _____

On the couch   _____

At the home computer   _____

Sitting eating meals   _____

Other   _____

Total sedentary debt per day: _____

How did you rate? It is not uncommon to score over 16, 17, 18, or even 19 hours per day. If you have a desk job, your number will be quite high. If you are on your feet most of the day, your score will be lower, giving you a slight health advantage over your fellow desk workers.

Even though standing does require more work than sitting, you will probably not be accessing your *full movement potential* during the day. Your full movement potential is defined as your body's current and untapped capabilities for balance, strength, flexibility, endurance, and coordination. This is explained in greater detail later in the chapter.

After totaling your sedentary debt score, find the group you fit into:

Group 1: 16+ hours

Chances are you have a desk job or sit a good portion of your day. For you, paying off your sedentary debt each day is essential to prevent your health account from losing funds.

This group may experience aches and pains and possibly weight gain. If you scored 19 or more—red alert! You could be on the verge of health bankruptcy.

Group 2: 14-16 hours

If you fit into this group you probably stand as much as you sit during the day. Although you have less sedentary debt than Group 1, you still need to pay attention to your health account.

Group 3: Less than 14 hours

Scoring here means you're quite active during your day, either at home or at work, and may even have a very physically demanding job such as a construction worker, mail carrier, supermom, etc.

Given the amount of movement, sedentary debt is not an issue—instead you need to focus on adding health dollars to your health account.

However, if you do have a physically demanding job, there is the possibility of overuse and imbalance of certain muscles. The recommendations at the end of this chapter will ensure your body stays healthy and free from injury in the years to come.

SEDENTARY DEBT IS NOT A PROBLEM

Sedentary debt is just like credit card debt. Using credit cards is okay as long as you pay off the balance at the end of each month. If you don't, you pay a price in the form of high interest.

Sedentary debt is the same. The debt is not the problem—what matters is whether or not you pay it off.

Later in this chapter you will learn how you can pay off your sedentary debt, as well as how you can add health dollars to your health account.

> *Sedentary debt is not the problem.*
> *What matters is whether or not you pay it off.*

THE MODERN LIFESTYLE

Consider this thought. How many hours per day do you think your great grandparents spent being sedentary? Compared to you, probably very few especially if you scored in Group 1 or 2. Your body is actually designed for the same purpose as your ancestors of 2000 years ago, yet you perform very different functions.

Modern day society is concerned about getting the most done with the least amount of physical effort. Vehicles, computers, remote controls, elevators, and escalators, make your life a breeze. There are even self-parking cars and robotic vacuums!

Today's lifestyle may save you time and energy, but your body pays the price.

> *Today's lifestyle may save you time and energy,*
> *but your body pays the price.*

YOUR POSTURAL ALIGNMENT

Your postural alignment is how your body is aligned in relation to the force of gravity. A well aligned body is balanced against gravity with all its major joints vertically and horizontally aligned. In this position, every movement operates efficiently and requires little effort to perform.

The photos below are of a patient who experienced severe back pain due to two herniated discs in the lower spine. The first photo shows the effects that high sedentary debt and health bankruptcy had on his posture. The second photo was taken after he replenished his health account with essential movement.

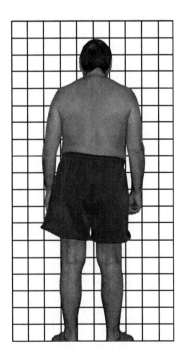

When the human frame is misaligned, it requires more energy to hold itself up. Aches and pains settle in and movements become difficult. The body becomes more susceptible to injury, fatigue, and arthritis.

Even conditions such as digestive problems and depression can be associated with misaligned posture.

When the body is misaligned, full movement potential is compromised.

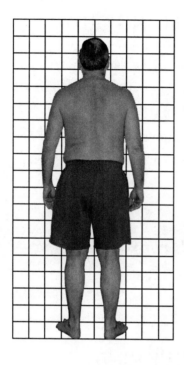

The aligned body is relaxed, at ease, and pain free. It is less susceptible to arthritis and injury.

Organs such as the heart, liver, kidneys, lungs, and intestines are in optimal position and function better. Energy flows through the acupuncture meridians more freely.

Full movement potential is optimized.

WHAT CAUSES MISALIGNED POSTURE?

Good posture deteriorates for many reasons. Injuries, surgeries, repetitive movements, underlying health conditions, and habitual mental/emotional states can cause misaligned posture. But the number one factor that contributes to the degradation of the human frame is *lack of use*.

The number one factor that contributes to the degradation of the human frame is lack of use.

ARE YOU REALLY "JUST GETTING OLD"?

People tend to become more sedentary and are inclined to do less and less as they get older. This isn't limited to individuals over 65—it can even apply to those in their 30's and 40's!

If you become less physically or mentally active as you age, the consequence is premature aging—and much of what is termed "aging" is merely the byproduct of neglect.

> *Much of what is termed "aging" is merely the byproduct of neglect.*

YOUTHFUL BODY, YOUTHFUL MIND

When introduced to new information, the body and mind stretch beyond their comfort zones to adapt and grow. A sure-fire way to slow the aging process is to implement new stimuli for growth.

My grandmother was a great example of this. She lived until she was 92 and remained mentally sharp as a whip until she passed on. I think a major reason for this was because she did crossword puzzles her whole life. The puzzles provided her brain with a challenging stimulus, forcing it to change and evolve.

The same principle applies to your body. It needs stimulating movements, fresh learning, and new experiences to keep it young.

You might even look and feel a bit younger than you did before you read this far! Joking aside, there is perhaps a hint of truth.

Your body needs stimulating movements, fresh learning, and new experiences to keep it young.

TAKING THE NEXT STEP

Here is a summary of what you've learned so far:

◊ Exercise as movement is the **first body essential to health and wellness.**

◊ Regular exercise increases strength, cardiovascular health, and helps to manage a healthy weight.

◊ The sedentary lifestyle is one of the biggest contributors to aging, postural misalignment, and increased susceptibility to injury, pain, and fatigue.

◊ Exercise is one of the secrets to the "fountain of youth". Longevity is maximized when you move your body.

◊ Specific health benefits of exercise are decreased risks of heart disease, cancer, diabetes, strokes, and osteoporosis among many others.

◊ Exercise can increase energy levels, improve mental clarity and mood. It also enhances your body's detoxification systems.

◊ Unpaid sedentary debt depletes your health account.

◊ Sedentary debt can be repaid and you can also add health dollars to your health account.

What do you do now?

First, pay off your sedentary debt. Second, add health dollars to your health account.

PAY OFF YOUR SEDENTARY DEBT

MOVE YOUR BODY FOR 15 MINUTES EACH DAY

If you are in Group 1 or 2, you need to move your body dynamically for at least 15 minutes every day to pay off your sedentary debt. In most cases, doing so will raise your score to neutral or zero in your health account.

Depending on your current level of health and ability, a dynamic exercise could be a brisk walk around the block or trail, a bike ride, a jog, or 15 minutes of yoga. Even dancing or raking leaves in your yard is considered dynamic exercise. It doesn't matter what you are doing as long as you are moving!

In the final section of this chapter you will create a plan to pay off your sedentary debt that includes the specific forms of movement you will perform daily. These days will be called your *regular days*.

Regular days are your daily deposits of movement into your health account. They pay off your sedentary debt.

Regular days pay off your sedentary debt.

If you are in Group 1 and have 19 or more hours of sedentary debt, you are in the red alert zone! This means you need to add at least 5 more minutes per day in order to get your body out of debt.

Just add the 5 minutes to the basic 15, or if you have time constraints, fit the extra 5 minutes in at another time of the day.

ADD HEALTH DOLLARS TO YOUR HEALTH ACCOUNT

CHALLENGE YOUR BODY FOR 15 MINUTES TWICE A WEEK

In order to add health dollars to your health account you need to kick it up a notch and *challenge* your body to move beyond its comfort zone at least twice a week.

This is essential if you are in Group 1 or 2, and a core requirement if you are in Group 3 and want to boost your health account.

Intensifying your workout makes your body more resilient, flexible, and robust. Your posture improves and your lungs and heart get stronger. Your metabolism and hormones are stimulated, making it easier to lose weight if desired.

Challenging your body also enhances your detoxification systems, as you will learn in Chapter 3.

> *To add health dollars to your health account, you need to challenge your body at least twice a week for at least 15 minutes.*

Choose an exercise that increases your heart rate, causes you to break a sweat, or creates some muscle burn.

Depending on your current fitness level, this could be as simple as adding an extra 15 minutes to your regular day 15 minute walk, and adding a block of jogging at the end.

You might want something more strenuous such as a 30 minute weight training workout or 20 minute bike ride twice a week. How about an hour of yoga or aquasize?

Sometimes a fast paced 15 minute run can be more challenging than a slow 30 minute bike ride. It depends on how hard you push yourself—you are the judge.

The bottom line is—if you are breathing hard, breaking a sweat, or your muscles are starting to burn, then you are pushing yourself.

If you are breathing hard, breaking a sweat, or your muscles are starting to burn, then you are pushing yourself.

These days are called your challenge days.

Challenge days develop your full movement potential, resulting in enhanced vitality and a health account brimming with an abundance of health dollars.

Challenge days take your health to a whole new level. They tap into and develop more of your full movement potential and add health dollars to your health account.

YOUR FULL MOVEMENT POTENTIAL

When I ask my patients about their exercise habits, the most common response I hear is: "I walk a lot."

Although walking is a beneficial foundation for regular days, it doesn't utilize your full movement potential, especially if you are physically capable for more.

Walking barely scratches the surface of most people's full movement potential because it is linear and limits your arms and legs to forward and backward motion. Additionally, the joints and muscles of your shoulders, elbows, wrists, hips, knees, ankles, and spine involve a very small range of motion.

Compare walking to activities like yoga, tai chi, or other martial arts where every joint of your body goes through a wide range of motion. The spine is bent, extended and twisted, the knees are fully flexed and straightened, the hips rotate, and the arms go overhead and even behind the back.

These are very dynamic practices that progress the whole body closer to its full movement potential.

TAPPING INTO YOUR FULL MOVEMENT POTENTIAL

Choose at least one other activity in addition to walking to enhance your full movement potential. Be creative. Do something that tests your body—something new, fresh, and dynamic. How about walking backwards for a few blocks to build your balance and coordination? You might get a few stares, but that could be as much fun as doing it!

> *Select at least one activity other than walking for your regular days or challenge days.*

Any activity that taps into and uses more of your body's full potential for balance, strength, flexibility, endurance, and coordination is the key. If you do not use these abilities, you will lose them.

If you are in Group 3 and spend many hours per day on your feet, consider an activity that uses your body in a new way like swimming, biking, strength training, or rowing. This maintains structural balance and reduces the effects of overuse. Adequate rest is also important.

SPECIAL CONSIDERATION FOR ACTIVE PEOPLE

If you are active and have a workout routine—great! However, there is always room to tap into your full movement potential by adding new forms of exercise.

If you do yoga, Pilates, or if you swim, try adding some weight training or running. Cross training taps into a wider range of balance, strength, flexibility, endurance, and coordination—components of a healthy balanced body.

Focusing only on areas where you excel may not necessarily be what you need. Try something new—your body will love you for it.

SELECTING MOVEMENT ACTIVITIES

There are a great variety of movement activities. Some focus on developing strength and endurance, while others improve flexibility, balance, and coordination.

Engaging in activities that work on all components is ideal but may be impractical if you are just getting started. Start by choosing one thing that you enjoy and go from there.

Here are a few possibilities for movement activities:

Very easy: Deep breathing, chair exercises, and gentle rehabilitative exercises.

Easy: Walking (forwards, backwards, and sideways), walk/running, dancing, stretching and limbering up exercises, and water exercises.

Challenging: Biking, jogging, yoga, tai chi and other martial arts, swimming, skiing, indoor climbing, fitness classes, fitness videos, strength training, skipping, rowing, and sports such as volleyball, tennis, soccer, and basketball.

As for sports, you don't have to join a team—just pick up a basketball and shoot a few hoops on your own or with a friend for 15 minutes.

A NOTE ON TREADMILLS

Walking or running outdoors is better for your biomechanics than using treadmills. When you place your foot down on a treadmill, it carries it backwards for you, but when you place your foot down on the earth, you have to push into the ground to propel your weight forward. The biomechanics are different. When possible, walk or run outdoors and enjoy the fresh air and sunshine too!

OTHER RECOMMENDATIONS FOR YOUR REGULAR DAYS AND CHALLENGE DAYS

◊   Enjoy what you are doing so it isn't merely a means to an end.

◊   Try something new (the anti-aging principle).

◊   Get outside! Fresh air and light have tremendous benefits, especially if you spend a lot of time indoors.

◊   Keep it local. It is easier to commit if you don't have to drive far.

◊   If you tend to be alone a lot, consider something social. If you are around people all the time, consider something on your own.

I highly recommend that children get involved in a sport or athletic activity while they are young and their bodies and minds are in development. Sports and exercise functionally develop the nervous system creating changes that will last throughout their lives.

SAMPLE PROGRAMS

Here are a few examples of weekly routines for the three groups that implement all of the principles you have learned:

GROUP 1: 16+ HOURS OF SEDENTARY DEBT

Example 1
5 regular days: brisk walking (15 min.)
2 challenge days: alternating walk/run (15 min.)

Example 2
5 regular days: brisk walking or tai chi video (15 min.)
2 challenge days: weight training (20 min.)

Example 3 (high sedentary debt of 19+ hours)
4 regular days: brisk walking at lunch (5 min.), brisk walking in the evening (15 min.)
3 challenge days: a mix of dancing, pushups, and jumping jacks (15 min. in total)

GROUP 2: 14–16 HOURS OF SEDENTARY DEBT

Example 1
5 regular days: brisk walking or easy bike ride (15 min.)
2 challenge days: yoga class 1 day (1 hr.), running 1 day (15 min.)

Example 2
5 regular days: brisk walking or yard work (15 min.)
2 challenge days: cardio kickboxing video (15 min.)

Example 3

4 regular days: brisk walking (30 min.)

3 challenge days: weight training 2 days (30 min.), hiking 1 day (30 min.)

GROUP 3: UNDER 14 HOURS OF SEDENTARY DEBT

Example 1

0 regular days: (job is physically demanding)

2 challenge days: swimming 1 day (25 min.), yoga 1 day (1 hr.)

Example 2

3 regular days: easy bike ride (15 min.)

2 challenge days: fitness video (15 min.)

Example 3

2 regular days: gentle yoga stretches (15 min.)

3 challenge days: running 2 days (15 min.), volleyball 1 day (1 hr.)

SUMMING UP

If you have already been paying off your sedentary debt each day, adding health dollars to your health account with challenge days, and are tapping into your full movement potential—congratulations! You have already mastered the **first body essential to health and wellness—** *movement*. Keep up the good work and move onto Chapter 2 to the **second body essential to health and wellness—***food*.

For everyone else, you are now going to put together your personalized program.

Get ready to awaken the health that has always been inside of you. The benefits are immediate and will last a lifetime. Have fun!

YOUR MOVEMENT ACTION PLAN

1. Write down every type of exercise, sport, or activity that you might like to try, even if it meant doing it only once.

   _____

   _____

   _____

2. Based on what you have learned from Chapter 1, write down 1, 2, or 3 movement activities that you will do for at least 15 minutes on your *regular days* each week. Next to each activity write down how many days and approximately how much time you will spend performing that activity in each session.

Regular Day Activity	No. of Days/Week	Time

3. Based on what you have learned from Chapter 1, write down 1, 2, or 3 movement activities that you will do for at least 15 minutes on your *challenge days* each week. Next to each activity write down how many days and approximately how much time you will spend performing that activity in each session.

Challenge Day Activity	No. of Days/Week	Time

4. Start your first regular day today!

5. Start your first challenge day this week!

Chapter (2)

FOOD

"Let your food be your medicine and your medicine be your food." These wise words were stated over 2000 years ago by the Greek physician Hippocrates, the father of modern medicine. His wisdom stands true today.

The fuel that you feed your body plays a vital role in preventing disease, maintaining a healthy weight, and helping you feel your best. As Hippocrates stated—food has the power to be your medicine.

Many common health problems from fatigue, aches and pains, digestive and hormonal problems to anxiety and depression can often improve by simply adjusting a few things in your diet.

Hence, the **second body essential of health and wellness—*food*.**

A HEALTHY DIET?

If you are confused by the dozens of fad diet and health books on the market, you're not alone.

Not only is the "one size fits all" approach to diet a myth, but much of the information available is contradictory. But beyond all the variables, there are some essential principles that should be a part of every diet. This chapter will explore these essential food principles to maximize your health, wellness, and longevity.

> *"Let your food be your medicine and your medicine be your food."*
>
> —Hippocrates

THE FOUNDATION: A WHOLE FOOD DIET

Naturally grown foods that are mostly unrefined, unprocessed and unpackaged, constitute a whole food diet—one of the most fundamental concepts of good nutrition.

However, the quality of food has substantially declined over the last few decades. Grocery store shelves are lined with all kinds of new packaged and processed "foods", environmental pollution and toxins have risen, and foods grown are lower in nutrients than they were just a few decades ago.[1,2] Fruits and vegetables that were once commonly grown organically are now sprayed with chemicals.

The single most important thing you can do to improve your health through diet is to follow a whole food regimen because these foods contain the highest amount of nutrients and the lowest amount of pollutants and toxic substances.

The concepts of whole foods and nutrition are explored in these three sections:

1. **The Top 6 Essentials**—the 6 most important diet concepts

2. **More Abundant Health**—going beyond The Top 6 Essentials

3. **Your Food Action Plan**—creating your personal health and wellness plan

The single most important thing you can do to improve your health through diet is to follow a whole food regimen.

THE TOP 6 ESSENTIALS

The Top 6 Essentials are the most important diet concepts that you need to implement for optimal health and wellness. They create a solid foundation of good nutrition from which you can build upon.

ESSENTIAL #1: ELIMINATE SUGAR

Sugar is the number one thing to *avoid* in your diet. It is not a whole food. Eliminating sugar from your diet (especially if you consume a lot) can dramatically improve your health. This not only includes white sugar but also hidden sugars in packaged foods containing high fructose corn syrup, dextrose, sucrose, glucose, fructose, and maltodextrin.

One study showed that the immune system's response dramatically decreases for up to 5 hours after consuming only 100 grams of sugar (about 2 cans of pop).[3]

Many health professionals consider excess dietary sugar to be one of the biggest contributors to an overgrowth of the fungus Candida albicans. This is a yeast that normally inhabits your intestines, but can grow out of control as a result of poor dietary habits, impaired digestion, low immunity, and certain medications such as antibiotics, antacids, cortisone, and birth control pills.[4-6]

Although medical science acknowledges that Candida albicans can be problematic for individuals with lowered immunity, women with vaginal yeast infections, and infants with thrush—it does not traditionally view it as a widespread problem. However, clinical results have proved otherwise. Many health practitioners have observed health improvements in patients that have taken dietary and therapeutic measures aimed at reducing yeast overgrowth in the body.[7,8]

An overgrowth of Candida has been associated with a wide range of health problems including gas, bloating, mental confusion, irritability, PMS, fatigue, behavior changes, and other conditions.[6,9] Some of these symptoms can be related to Candida having produced alcohol as a toxic byproduct in the body.[6]

One of the keys to eliminating Candida overgrowth is to stop providing the yeast with its main source of fuel—sugar. All forms of sugar as well as alcohol and refined white flour act as fertilizers for Candida yeast.[5,10]

> *Sugar is the number one thing to avoid in your diet.*

Sugar has so many health problems related to it that the list is overwhelming and nearly endless.[11]

If you want to use sweeteners, there are many optional, more wholesome choices such as raw unpasteurized honey, maple syrup, blackstrap molasses, or organic unrefined cane sugar. Dates can also be used as a sweetener in hot cereals and baking. Although these sources provide a balance of vitamins, minerals, and other nutrients, they should still be used in small amounts. (Do not give honey to children under 1 year.)

Another excellent healthy sweetener is stevia, derived from a plant native to Paraguay. Stevia is hundreds of times sweeter than sugar and has virtually no calories. It may also be one of the few sweeteners that does not feed Candida. Unrefined stevia is green in colour and still contains its vitamins, minerals, and phytonutrients making it the preferred choice. Green stevia also tastes better than the refined white variety. Stevia can be found in most health food stores.

You may want to do a little research on how to bake with these sweeteners, but they can all be used to create delicious treats.

Many diet products often contain chemical sweeteners such as aspartame, sucralose, or saccharin. While artificial sweeteners are low in calories, they contain no nutritional value and some studies have shown these chemicals to be potentially linked with adverse health effects.[12-14] The long term consequences of using them are unknown, so it's best to avoid them.

ESSENTIAL #2: VEGETABLES

Yes, you guessed right. Vegetables are the top priority item to *increase* in your diet. They provide your body with abundant vitamins, minerals, phytonutrients, fiber, enzymes, and vital life energy rarely found in other foods. Yet, many people eat far too little of these life-giving essentials.

Aim to make vegetables an essential part of your lunch and dinner. Focus on boosting your intake of nutrient rich leafy greens such as kale, Swiss chard, broccoli, collard greens, mustard greens, and spinach. Not only are they packed with nutrients, they also provide the often lacking bitter flavour in the diet which is beneficial for the liver.

Including other coloured vegetables in your diet such as orange varieties (squash, yams, carrots), and purple veggies (eggplant, onions, cabbage) will give you a broad spectrum of phytonutrients.

Some of the less common vegetables to integrate into your diet for their specific health benefits include: artichoke for the liver/gallbladder, sea vegetables (known as seaweeds) such as kelp, dulse, and kombu for boosting mineral levels, and unpasteurized sauerkraut for providing healthy bacteria in your gut.

Although consuming raw vegetables does provide the highest nutrient value, eating too many can irritate the colon and weaken your digestion. Lightly steamed, stir fried or baked are a better choice for regular consumption. (Refer to Essential #4: *Eating with the Seasons* for more information on choosing and preparing.)

> *Vegetables are the top priority item to increase in your diet.*

ESSENTIAL #3: WHOLE GRAINS

White flour (breads, crackers, muffins, etc.), white pasta, white rice, and processed cereals are a common part of the traditional North American diet, yet these foods are highly processed and devoid of many nutrients. Whole grains should make up the majority of your carbohydrate intake as they are more nutrient dense and contain lots of healthy fiber.

The most familiar grains are wheat, oats, and rye, but there are also other healthy whole grains you can add to your diet. Try introducing brown rice, spelt, kamut, buckwheat, wild rice, millet, and quinoa. These grains have unique tastes and nutritional benefits.

Quinoa (pronounced keen-wa) is highly nutritious, easy to digest and quick to cook. It is also gluten-free. Quinoa makes a delicious side dish—try adding a little flax oil, olive oil, or butter. Use it where you would normally have rice, pasta, or potatoes.

These grains are available in their whole grain form or as flours, pastas, breads, and cereals and can be purchased at most health food stores.

If you need to lose weight, it is absolutely necessary to eliminate refined, processed flours and grains and introduce small to moderate amounts of high quality whole grains. Whole grains keep your blood sugar more stable than refined grains and flours, and are also packed with nutrients. Some people do even better by avoiding all grains entirely.

> *Try introducing brown rice, spelt, kamut, buckwheat,*
> *wild rice, millet, and quinoa.*

WHEAT SENSITIVITY

Wheat is the most commonly consumed grain in the North American diet, yet unbeknownst to many, is also one of the most common food sensitivities.

Wheat sensitivity can cause a number of symptoms such as mental fogginess, fatigue, skin problems (eczema, acne), and digestive symptoms such as bloating, diarrhea, and constipation.

However, wheat sensitivity should not be confused with Celiac disease which is a more serious condition where one is intolerant to the gluten found in wheat and other grains.

Food sensitivities are akin to minor allergies. When you stop eating foods that you are sensitive to, your health often improves.

If you think you might be sensitive to wheat, try avoiding it for two weeks and monitor how you feel. Begin using some of the alternative grains mentioned above or try sprouted wheat bread.

Many people are sensitive to wheat without realizing it.

SPROUTED WHEAT BREAD

Sprouted wheat breads are made from sprouted grain—not flour. During the sprouting process, grains break down and "predigest" thereby improving digestibility. Phytic acid, which can impair mineral absorption, is also decreased during the sprouting process.

This is the same reason why it's important to soak beans before cooking. Soaking starts the sprouting process which reduces phytic acid and makes the beans easier to digest.

Some sprouted wheat breads are lighter and easier to digest than many whole grain breads. If you are sensitive to wheat or have difficulties digesting bread, you may find Ezekiel 4:9® brand sprouted wheat bread or wraps to be a good alternative. It can be found in some grocery and health food stores in the freezer section.

ESSENTIAL #4: EATING WITH THE SEASONS

Traditional Chinese medicine states that eating locally grown foods that are in season support the body to harmoize with its environment. One fundamental principle is that foods are seen to have a *warming* or *cooling* effect on your body, depending upon the type of food you consume and how it is prepared.

For example, in the heat of the summer your body can benefit from the cooling effect of fresh fruit and summer vegetables, whereas in the winter your body benefits more from the warming effect of cooked foods like soups and stews—especially those made with winter root vegetables like squash, turnips, rutabaga, and sweet potatoes.

When you eat fruits and vegetables that are locally grown and in season, their natural properties help keep your body in energetic and physiological balance with the environment.

This principle is most important in the consumption and preparation of fruit and vegetables but can also be applied to other foods such as meats, spices, and grains.

When you eat fruits and vegetables that are locally grown and in season, their natural properties help keep your body in balance with its environment.

HOW TO KEEP YOUR DIGESTION STRONG

Healthy digestion supports all systems in your body including your muscles and bones, hormones, circulation, immune system, and mental/emotional wellness.

Your digestive tract constitutes up to 80% of your immune system, and because of its unique intricate nervous system, some researchers call it your "second brain".[15]

Traditional Chinese medicine compares your digestive system to a bubbling pot on a stove, with the flame of the stove being the strength or fire of digestion. If you put a lot of cooling foods (see list below) into the pot (your stomach), your body's "digestive fire" can be put out, resulting in a weakened digestive system. This can lead to symptoms such as gas, bloating, yeast overgrowth, aches and pains, fatigue, a tendency to feel cold, lowered immunity, and other health problems.

Since your digestion feeds your whole system, any part of your body can be affected if it goes off kilter. The opposite is also true—if it is working smoothly, any health problem can be improved.

FOODS THAT ARE COOLING

◊   fruits and raw vegetables (especially banana and melon)

◊   fruit and vegetable juices (very cooling)

◊   tofu, soy milk, and bean sprouts

◊   refrigerated foods and drinks, frozen foods (ice cream, popsicles, ice water, etc.)

FOODS THAT ARE WARMING

◊ cooked foods in general

◊ most protein foods—meats, fish, eggs, beans (especially black beans)

◊ whole grains, nuts and seeds

◊ healthy oils and butter

Digestive fire can also be aggravated by too many very warm or "hot" foods such as coffee, hot spices, alcohol, and deep fried foods.

Adding warming spices such as garlic, ginger, black pepper, cumin, coriander, turmeric, nutmeg, and cinnamon to cooling foods, can warm them up to a degree.

Naturopathic physician, Dr. Jonn Matsen, suggests that adding unrefined sea salt to cooked vegetables can warm them up more by increasing sodium levels in relation to potassium. He found that the body requires higher levels of sodium when vitamin D levels are low from lack of sun exposure, and that too much potassium (fruit and veggies) and not enough sodium in the winter can cause digestive weakness. (Vitamin D is needed to help your body absorb calcium.)

Therefore, in the cooler weather, be sure to add unrefined sea salt to your cooked veggies to increase warming properties. (Technically, most cooked vegetables are classified as cooling, but are warming in relation to raw.)

If you have a robust digestion and live in a hot climate, you can usually consume larger amounts of raw fruits and vegetables and other cooling foods without a problem. Summer-like weather may be year round or only for a couple of months of the year, depending on where you live.

Cooling foods may be therapeutically indicated for some people with a strong "hot" constitution or condition, but a diet that leans to the warming side is preferred for most. (For a description of the hot constitution/condition, refer to the end of Chapter 3: *Selecting a Detoxification Method*.)

This doesn't mean you need to avoid all raw food. Just eat it in moderation, especially in cooler weather or if you have digestive problems.

Here are the key points to keeping your digestion healthy and strong:

◊   Don't overeat cooling foods.

◊   Lightly cook most foods, especially during the cooler months.

◊   Try to eat foods that are local and in season.

◊   Use unrefined sea salt on your veggies, especially in cooler weather.

ESSENTIAL #5: ORGANICALLY GROWN FOOD

The jury is in—organically grown food tastes better, is higher in nutritional value, isn't genetically engineered, and doesn't contribute to polluting your body or the planet with chemicals.[16-20] Try to make organically grown food a regular part of your diet.

There are some issues to be aware of with animal products. Non-organic animal products are often filled with growth hormones, antibiotics, pesticides, colouring agents, and other pollutants. These substances accumulate in the animals' bodies and are then passed on to yours.

Unfortunately, even wild fish are contaminated with increasing levels of mercury (industrial pollution), polychlorinated biphenyls (PCBs), and other pollutants.[21] The results of this were recently seen in killer whales off the coast of British Columbia in Canada, which were found to have incredibly high levels of PCBs in their bodies.[22] These animals feast on fish and sea mammals.

If you eat animal products, organically fed, hormone free, antibiotic free, and free-range raised animals provide the best choice for you, the animals, and the planet. With fish, smaller, younger fish contain the least amount of contaminants, whereas older, larger, and carnivorous fish such as shark, some types of tuna, king mackerel (king fish), tilefish, and swordfish contain higher levels of toxins (especially mercury) that have accumulated over time.

At the time of this writing, Health Canada indicates that the following fish are considered low in mercury and safe to eat: anchovy, capelin, char, hake, herring, Atlantic mackerel, mullet, pollock (Boston bluefish), salmon, smelt, rainbow trout, lake whitefish, blue crab, shrimp, clam, mussel, oyster, and some types of tuna.[23]

At present, some types of canned tuna are considered to have acceptable amounts of mercury. Yellowfin, tongol, and light tuna have relatively low mercury levels with *skipjack* being the lowest.[24] Albacore is higher and bluefin is one of the highest. However, albacore caught off the coast of British Columbia are younger and considerably lower in mercury than older albacore from southern waters. Bluefin tuna is often used in sushi and should be avoided.[24]

Although considered "acceptable", mercury levels in canned tuna are significantly higher than canned salmon, making salmon the preferred health choice.[25] Salmon is also higher in omega 3 fatty acids. Pink salmon is the overall best choice because they mature within 2 years, leaving little time to build up toxins.

The U.S. FDA states that young children, and women who are breastfeeding, pregnant or planning on becoming pregnant, should not consume high level mercury fish and should avoid eating *any* seafood more than twice per week.[26]

Unless organically fed, farmed fish *do not* provide a better option as they contain even higher contaminants than wild fish.[27]

Avoid the skin in fish as it tends to store higher levels of toxins.

Make organically grown food a regular part of your diet.

ESSENTIAL #6: FRESH LOCALLY GROWN FOOD

Locally grown foods do not have to travel long distances before arriving on your dinner plate. This means that fresh fruits and vegetables are picked much closer to ripening, taste better and are nutritionally superior. Farmers' markets often provide the best quality of fresh, locally grown produce, meats and other products.

BUYING LOCAL AND THE ENVIRONMENT

Buying locally grown food also reduces your personal environmental footprint because less transport means fewer emissions.

The air you breathe, the soil your food grows in, and the water you drink come from the environment. Good health relies on the quality and purity of these natural elements. These elements can be viewed as extensions of your own individual body or perhaps you as extensions of them. From this perspective, the obvious course of action is to choose foods that support both your body and the planet's body.

Buying locally grown food reduces your personal environmental footprint on the planet.

MORE ABUNDANT HEALTH

If you feel comfortable with The Top 6 Essentials and are ready to take your health and wellness to the next level, this section will explore how to implement healthy whole foods on all fronts. For those who found The Top 6 Essentials to be sufficient for now, you might consider adding just one suggestion from this section to *Your Food Action Plan* at the end of this chapter. You can always revisit this chapter later when you feel ready.

SALT

Common refined table salt is stripped of nearly all its trace minerals. Whole *unrefined* sea salt is often grey in colour and contains a balance of minerals beyond sodium chloride. Use this salt in all your cooking and seasoning. Unrefined sea salt can be purchased in most health food stores, and should not be confused with sea salts found in most grocery stores—most of which are refined and similar to table salt.

Since most unrefined sea salts lack iodine, it is advised to use seaweeds such as kelp, dulse, kombu, wakame, and hijiki in your diet. They are all high in iodine which is needed for proper thyroid function. Small amounts of kelp or dulse flakes can be sprinkled on vegetables and strips of whole seaweed such as kombu can be added to stews, soups, beans, etc. These sea vegetables also contain a spectrum of other minerals, vitamins, and nutrients. Other sources of iodine include dairy products (especially yogurt), eggs, strawberries, and seafood. Sushi rolls wrapped in seaweed, provide another source.

DAIRY

Dairy, including milk, cheese, and butter are common diet staples and contain valuable fats, protein, vitamins, and minerals such as calcium. However, the problem with cow dairy is that many people are either lactose intolerant, allergic to the protein in milk (casein), or sensitive to cow dairy in general.

DAIRY SENSITIVITY

Dairy sensitivity can cause a spectrum of symptoms such as digestive problems, skin problems, and fatigue. If you suspect you or your child are sensitive to dairy from cows, try eliminating it for 2 weeks and observe any improvements.

Cultured or fermented dairy products such as yogurt and kefir are generally easier to digest because casein protein and lactose breaks down during the fermenting process. Fermenting also adds enzymes and friendly bacteria. Be sure to buy a quality organic brand such as Stonyfield Farm®, or make your own to ensure active bacterial cultures are present in significant amounts. Some brands state that they contain "live and active cultures" which is ideal. Although all yogurts are *made* with active cultures, they may not still contain them as these bacteria are killed off in the pasteurization process.

Goat's milk is a good alternative to cow's milk as it is easier to digest because it contains less casein and lactose, and no agglutinin.

Rice milk, soy milk, almond milk, and hemp seed milk are also good alternatives and usually fortified with vitamins A, D, and calcium.

(Not to be used as replacements for breast milk or infant formula in children under the age of 2.)

Soy milk should only be consumed in small amounts. It is high in phytates which block mineral absorption in the body, is high in phytoestrogens which alter hormones, and is very cooling to the body. Like dairy and wheat, soy is a common food sensitivity.

Eating small amounts of whole fat or two percent dairy is better than large amounts of low fat products. Your body needs the fat to stabilize blood sugar levels and assist in the absorption of other nutrients.

Also, avoid margarine—use butter instead. Margarine is a manufactured, processed product—not a whole food.

In addition to dairy products, other good sources of calcium are found in sesame seeds, canned salmon with bones, broccoli, beans, almonds, and most green leafy veggies. While spinach, chard, and beet greens do contain calcium, these foods also contain oxalate and phytate which reduce calcium absorption.

> *Other good sources of calcium are found in sesame seeds, canned salmon with bones, broccoli, beans, almonds, and most green leafy vegetables.*

FRUIT

Fruit is high in fiber, vitamins, and minerals, but is also a cooling food and can weaken the digestive system if overeaten. Enjoy in moderation.

If you live in a colder climate, eat fresh fruit when it is in season during summer and early fall, and small amounts of non-tropical fruits during the off-season. Some of the best fruits to eat year round are berries—blueberries, cranberries, blackberries, and raspberries. They are lower in sugars and packed with phytonutrients. Other good options for the cooler seasons are small amounts of cooked fruits such as apple sauce and fruit cobblers made with healthy sweeteners.

Remember to primarily eat fruit grown locally in your area if possible.

Cooking fruit with warming spices such as cardamom, ginger, cinnamon, or nutmeg helps balance the cooling energy of fruit by adding a warming energy. These spices are also helpful for digestion.

FRUIT JUICE

Fruit juice is very sweet and also cooling. It should not be consumed in large amounts on a regular basis. Dilute juices with water, especially for children.

> *Fruit juice is very sweet and cooling. It should not be consumed in large amounts on a regular basis.*

FATS AND OILS

Fats, including oils, are an important part of your diet. They provide essential fatty acids, assist in metabolism, enhance the immune system and vitamin absorption, create the foundation for hormone production, and act as a source of calories. Fat has acquired a bad rap, but the reality is that your body requires an abundance of healthy fat in your daily diet.

Here are a few recommendations:

◊ Be sure to use only organic *unrefined* oils. These oils taste better, have not been chemically processed, and retain more nutrients such as antioxidants (vitamin E, carotenes), phytosterols, chlorophyll, lecithin, and others.[28]

◊ Avoid low quality refined oils like refined corn, safflower, soybean, canola, etc.

◊ Frying destroys all oils but some less than others.[29] The best fats and oils to use for high temperature cooking are organic coconut oil, butter, and ghee (clarified butter).[29] If you must use other oils for frying, *refined* oils are preferred as they withstand high temperatures better than unrefined oils. Refined peanut oil, sesame oil, and grapeseed oil are the best options.[29] Avoid deep fried foods.

◊ To prevent deterioration and rancidity, most oils are best stored in the fridge with the exception of coconut oil and ghee. Although olive oil is best refrigerated, it thickens. Storing it in a cool, dark place will suffice. Be sure to buy oils packaged in dark glass containers.

◊ Avoid all hydrogenated and partially hydrogenated oils found in shortening and packaged foods. They produce trans-fatty acids which increase "bad" cholesterol, create inflammation in the body, negatively affect the immune system, and contribute to diseases such as diabetes, heart disease, and strokes.[30]

◊ Many animal products (cheese, butter, eggs, and meats) are high in saturated fats, which in moderation are beneficial to the body. Simply choose lean cuts of meat, and balance your meals with plenty of vegetables to assist digestion and provide complimentary nutrients.

OMEGA 3 FATTY ACIDS

Omega 3 fatty acids play a vital role in your immune system, cardiovascular system, hormonal system, brain and nervous system—essentially your whole body. Since fish is the best source of these essential fatty acids, try to eat low mercury varieties such as salmon, twice a week. Other less potent sources of omega 3's are flaxseeds and walnuts.

Omega 3 fatty acids are especially important for women who are pregnant or breastfeeding, and young children because they are crucial in the health and development of the brain and nervous system. Even women who are intending to get pregnant should ensure they are getting adequate omega 3's *before* they get pregnant as these fats play a crucial role in the initial developmental processes of the fetus, particularly the nervous system.

Since these groups are also the most susceptible to the effects of mercury toxicity, fish oil supplements should be considered.

ANIMAL PRODUCTS

Meat and poultry provide high sources of protein. If you eat meat, choose lean cuts from organically raised animals. Even better, aim to find meat and dairy products from grass fed cows. Cows fed their natural diet of grass—as opposed to grain—produce meat and milk that is nutritionally superior. Specifically it is higher in omega 3 fatty acids.

If you are a meat eater, integrate some vegetarian meals into your diet each week to balance your diet with nutrients from other protein sources such as beans, lentils, and tofu. Also, because raising livestock requires more water, land, and fossil fuel than grains and vegetables, you help protect the environment when you consume less meat.[31]

(For information on fish see Essential #5: *Organically Grown Food* and More Abundant Health: *Fats and Oils*.)

> *Integrate some vegetarian meals each week to balance your diet with other protein sources such as beans, lentils, and tofu.*

Eggs are also an excellent food choice because they are high in protein and contain a wide range of vitamins, minerals, and other nutrients such as omega 3 and 6 fatty acids. They also contain choline—a nutrient that supports your nervous system. Other good souces of choline include beef, cauliflower, tofu, almonds, and peanuts.

Since the cooking process decreases nutrient levels in eggs, poaching or soft boiling are the best cooking methods.[32]

NUTS AND SEEDS

Nuts and seeds are high in vitamin E and essential fatty acids, however they tend to turn rancid fairly quickly after being shelled. Keep them in the refrigerator to protect their oils. Ideally, choose organic nuts and seeds that are sold in coolers, available in some health food stores.

Nuts are very rich and traditional Chinese medicine states they congest the liver and gallbladder. If you have symptoms of PMS, high blood pressure, menopause, a red tongue with yellow coat, or are easily angered—all signs of liver congestion—you should avoid or limit nuts.

If you eat peanut butter, buy brands that do not contain hydrogenated oils or sugar. Almond butter, pumpkin seed butter, cashew butter, and mixed nut butters provide a balance of other nutrients not found in peanut butter. (Peanut is actually a legume, not a nut.)

> *Nuts and seeds should be stored in the refrigerator to protect their oils.*

BEANS AND LENTILS

Beans and lentils are a part of the legume family. They contain essential fatty acids and high amounts of protein, B-vitamins and minerals—calcium, magnesium, potassium, zinc, selenium, and iron. Beans and lentils are an excellent protein alternative to meat.

There are a wide variety to choose from—aduki, black beans, black-eyed peas, garbanzo, kidney beans, lentils, lima, mung beans, navy beans, peas, pinto, and soybeans (including tofu).

Tofu is quite versatile for cooking and fairly easy to digest, but is cold in nature and should be cooked with warming spices such as ginger, garlic, and cumin. Tofu is best used in small amounts or eaten infrequently as it is high in glutamate and has been linked with decreased brain function.[33]

Legumes are most easily digested when eaten with green leafy or non-starchy vegetables. If you are cooking dried beans, make sure to soak them first for about 12 hours or overnight (less time for smaller beans) to improve cooking and digestibility. Rinse them and use fresh water before cooking and scoop the foam off when simmering.

Adding a strip of seaweed such as kombu during soaking and cooking can further aid digestion and adds extra minerals—especially iodine. If using salt, add at the end of cooking to avoid hardening the beans.

THERAPEUTIC BENEFITS OF BEANS AND LENTILS

According to traditional Chinese medicine, beans—especially aduki beans and black beans—are beneficial to the kidneys and adrenal glands.

Recent research has shown black beans to be extremely high in antioxidants, containing approximately as much as grapes and cranberries, and 10 times that of oranges.[34]

The kidneys are considered to be the root of one's life energy, and are weak in many people. Common symptoms of kidney weakness in traditional Chinese medicine include low energy, low back pain, knee pain, frequent urination, hair loss, poor memory, depression, fear, and insecurity. High stress, poor nutrition, lack of exercise, and fears and insecurities are prominent causes of kidney and adrenal weakness.

Liver imbalances are often associated with kidney weakness and can be improved by addressing the factors previously mentioned along with resolving the liver emotions which are anger and frustration.

BEVERAGES

Drinking adequate water is important but the amount varies for each individual. Your requirements will change based on your activity levels, diet, and lifestyle. A reasonable average for most people is 6–8 glasses per day.

Some people take the "drink water" advice to an extreme and guzzle it all day long—don't overdo it. Drinking too much water puts a strain on your kidneys and can deplete your mineral levels.

Be sure to drink good quality filtered water. Traditional Chinese medicine advises against drinking cold water as it can weaken digestion by putting out the digestive fire. Drink it at room temperature.

> *Traditional Chinese medicine advises against drinking cold water as it can weaken digestion.*
> *Drink it at room temperature.*

Herbal teas are another good beverage choice, some with specific health benefits. The quality and taste varies dramatically between brands. Enjoy a good quality organic tea—they are much tastier.

Here are a few good choices along with their corresponding health benefits:

◊   roiboos tea – antioxidant, liver support, anti-cancer

◊   tulsi tea (holy basil) – antioxidant and anti-stress

◊   green tea – antioxidants and liver support

◊   licorice tea – beneficial to the adrenal glands

◊   ginger tea – digestive aid and anti-nausea

◊   peppermint tea – digestive aid and calming

◊   dandelion tea – digestive aid and detoxifying properties[35]

Be sure to choose organic teas to avoid infusing pesticides at the same time.

WHAT TO AVOID

Avoid coffee, pop, alcohol, refined sugar, fast food, artificial flavors and colours, and artificial sweeteners as they have little, if any nutritional value and can create health problems. Occasional consumption is okay as long as you don't include them as a regular part of your diet.

I have seen dramatic health improvements in some of my patients after they simply eliminated their daily coffee intake. Coffee stimulates stress hormones from the adrenal glands and can contribute to adrenal exhaustion—a common state if you are overstressed and overworked.[36] It also congests the liver.

Lastly, avoid microwave ovens. Studies have shown that cooking food in a microwave oven decreases nutrient levels and creates changes in the food which can negatively impact your physiology.[37,38] Use your stove and oven.

FOOD COMBINING

To keep blood sugar levels balanced, ensure each meal contains a serving of a protein (meat, beans, eggs, cheese, etc.), a carbohydrate (grains, veggies, etc.), and some healthy fats (olive oil, butter, nuts/ seeds, etc.).

Because fruit is high in natural sugars, it digests easiest when eaten apart from most other foods, especially protein. The combination of sugar and protein in the digestive tract causes fermentation which can produce gas, bloating, and digestive weakness. If you have a blood sugar imbalance, you may prefer to eat protein with fruit.

EATING HABITS

Remember the basics:

◊   Avoid habitual overeating.

◊   Chew your food well.

◊   Be present when you eat and avoid distractions.

◊   Avoid eating late or just before bed. Your body needs to rest and detoxify during the night—not be overburdened with digesting.

SUPPLEMENTATION

In an ideal state of perfect health with a high quality whole food diet, a non-toxic environment, and a balanced emotional life—dietary supplementation would not be necessary. But the reality is that most of us have some level of health imbalance, live in a toxic environment, are often stressed, and rarely eat optimally with consistency. Therefore some supplementation is recommended as a healthy adjunct to a whole food diet.

As well, the level of nutrients in food has declined over the last few decades due to high yield crops and chemical sprays.[1,2] Low dietary levels of vitamins A, C, E, calcium, magnesium, potassium, and fiber have also been found in the general public.[39] We are an overfed and undernourished population.

While dietary supplements can be used as an adjunct to enhance nutrition, vibrant health is derived from implementing long term, good eating habits.

> *Vibrant health is derived from implementing long term, good eating habits.*

THE TOP 3 SUPPLEMENTS

The following 3 supplements will fill any gaps in your diet and support your body's essential processes. Although there is a plethora of useful supplements on the market, I consider these to be fundamental.

Take these 3–6 days per week.

HIGH QUALITY MULTIVITAMIN

A high quality multivitamin is a good base to ensure you are getting a spectrum of nutrients—some of which you may either be missing in your diet or not metabolizing properly. Be sure to use a product that is in capsule form—not tablet. Capsules are easier to digest and do not contain binders.

HIGH QUALITY FISH OIL SUPPLEMENT

As discussed in *Fats and Oils*, the omega 3 essential fats that are contained in fish support your whole body—your immune system, hormonal system, cardiovascular system, brain and nervous system.

Unless you eat fish twice per week, a high quality fish oil supplement taken periodically will ensure you are getting sufficient omega 3's. Look for brands that have been "molecularly distilled" to ensure purity and integrity. Children, and women who are breast feeding or pregnant, or intending to get pregnant, should also take fish oil to reap the benefits of omega 3 fats while avoiding the potential toxins in fish.

PROBIOTIC SUPPLEMENT

A world of microbes known as *digestive flora* are living in your digestive tract. These microbes consist of both healthy bacteria which aid digestion, as well as unhealthy microorganisms such as harmful bacteria and yeast.

Stress, unhealthy eating, and environmental toxins can contribute to an imbalance in your digestive flora causing the yeast and harmful bacteria to outnumber the "good" bacteria.

You can support the good bacteria in your digestive tract by periodically taking a supplement that contains the healthy bacterial strains *L. acidophilus* and *bifidobacterium*—commonly known as "probiotics". These bacteria support your digestive and immune systems by keeping the harmful microorganisms from overpopulating.

Food sources of these healthy bacteria strains include quality yogurt, kefir, unpasteurized sauerkraut, kimchii, umeboshi plums, unpasteurized miso, and unpasteurized milk. Unless you eat these foods on a regular basis, include a probiotic supplement into your regular regime.

Probiotic supplements are especially recommended after taking antibiotics and when travelling to countries where food hygiene may be a concern.

Take probiotic supplements with food.

OTHER CONSIDERATIONS

FOLIC ACID

Women intending to get pregnant are advised to take a supplement containing folic acid in order to prevent birth defects.

VITAMIN B12

Since vitamin B12 is primarily found in animal products, strict vegetarian diets are likely to be B12 deficient. If meat, eggs, or dairy are not a staple in your diet, be sure to supplement with this nutrient. Use a sublingual (under the tongue) B12 tablet or liquid to ensure effective absorption. If you are over age 50, you may also benefit from extra vitamin B12 as stomach acid tends to diminish with age and is required for vitamin B12 absorption. People taking antacids or antiulcer medication should also add this supplement.

VITAMIN D

If you live in a climate where there is a lot of cloudy weather and/or spend considerable time indoors, or if you are over age 50, be sure to supplement with extra vitamin D. Vitamin D plays a vital role in calcium absorption, bone health, and immunity. Because your body is able to create its own vitamin D when exposed to the ultraviolet rays from the sun, be sure to get outside daily even if it is just for a few minutes.

INDIVIDUAL CONCERNS

Nutritional supplements can also be used to treat specific health conditions, but for this purpose should be supervised by a health care professional. Taking one vitamin or nutrient in large doses can upset the metabolism of other nutrients—and what may be good for one person may be useless or even harmful to another.

To revisit the words of Hippocrates—"Let your food be your medicine and your medicine be your food".

> *"Let your food be your medicine and your medicine be your food."*

LISTEN TO YOUR BODY

Your dietary needs are not static. They can change by the day, the week or the season. Be mindful and listen to your body. It will guide you to make wise food choices. Avoid the extremes of emotional eating or strict regimens.

By implementing the information in this chapter you can begin to make gradual, positive changes to your eating habits that will benefit all aspects of your life.

And remember—it's what you do most of the time that really matters.

Now get ready to give your body a major boost by creating your health and wellness plan, and putting it into action. Let's do it!

YOUR FOOD ACTION PLAN

1. **Sugars**
   Which foods containing sugars do you regularly consume that you will eliminate or reduce in your diet? _____
   _____
   _____

2. **Vegetables**
   List three green vegetables that you will buy the next time you get groceries. How will you prepare them? Steamed, baked, stir fried, or a specific recipe? Commit to eating your veggies daily. _____
   _____

3. **Whole Grains**
   Write down one or more wheat alternative grain(s) (brown rice pasta, spelt bread, quinoa grain, etc.) that you will buy the next time you get groceries. If you're not sure, browse the health food store/section for options. Commit to reducing your intake of refined white flour starting today. _____
   _____

4. **Eating Seasonally**
   Are there any fruits or raw veggies that you routinely eat a lot of when they are out of season? If so, what is a better option?
   _____
   _____

5. **Buying Locally Grown**
   "I will find out where my food is produced and if possible will choose locally grown alternatives." (check) ☐

6. **Organic Food**
   If you are not currently eating organic food, what level of commitment do you want to make—a total switch to organic or just a few foods? If just a few foods, what are they?
   _____
   _____

7. **More Abundant Health**
   Are there any other food or dietary habits that you want to start implementing right now? If so, what are they?

   _____

   _____

   _____

   _____

   _____

   _____

Chapter (3)

DETOXIFICATION

CAVEAT

Before starting this chapter, I invite you to first adopt a specific mind set—one that holds the belief that you are healthy. After reading through the list of toxins that you are exposed to in your daily life, you might feel that the world is a dangerous place and that you are at the mercy of health robbing toxins wherever you go.

While it is necessary and wise to take action to improve your health—living in fear is neither helpful nor healthy. Beliefs have the power to control your physiology (as you will learn in *Book 2: Mind*), and create health or disease—regardless of your environment.

So if you are willing, first adopt the belief that you are healthy and then do the things that support this belief.

> *First adopt the belief that you are healthy, and then do the things that support this belief.*

Your body is remarkable. Every second, billions of functions are occurring, each one playing a key role to maintain health. This natural tendency for your body to self-regulate is called homeostasis—an innate ability to balance and adapt to various stresses in life—physical, mental, or emotional.

If any stress becomes too great for your body to handle, signs or symptoms will manifest. One form of physical stress is environmental toxins.

ENVIRONMENTAL TOXINS

Environmental toxins are chemicals and substances that come from any outside source—the air you breathe, the water your drink, the food you ingest, or physical contact and absorption through your skin. Environmental toxins are harmful to the health of the body/mind system and contribute to your toxic burden level.

Examples of environmental toxins are toxic metals (primarily mercury, lead, cadmium, aluminum, and arsenic), pesticides, DDT, food additives, phthalates (plastics), formaldehyde, fire retardants, fumes from non-stick coatings[1], stain repellents, and chemicals such as PCBs (polychlorinated biphenyls). These are just a few of the thousands of different toxins that you are exposed to in today's world.

YOUR BODY'S TOXIC BURDEN LEVEL

Your toxic burden level is the cumulation of all toxic substances that your body is currently holding and dealing with. Each of us will have different burden levels depending on exposure history and health status, but studies confirm that likely everyone carries a load of dozens of chemicals and toxins in their body.[2,3]

Even fetuses and infants can be exposed to high levels of toxins as they are passed directly through the umbilical blood and mother's breast milk.[4-6]

> *Your toxic burden level is the cumulation of all toxic substances that your body is currently dealing with.*

TOXINS AND YOUR HEALTH

Toxic chemicals and pollutants can alter proper functioning of your immune system, hormonal system, and nervous system.[2] They can cause a wide range of physical, mental or emotional symptoms ranging from asthma, allergies, and mood changes to autoimmune disease, cancer, and neurological problems.[2]

INTERNAL TOXINS

Your body naturally produces some toxins as byproducts of metabolism. Organisms that live inside the body such as yeast, bacteria, and parasites are also capable of producing toxins. These internal toxins are easily managed when healthy but can create health issues if you are too sedentary, not eating well, emotionally stressed, or when your toxic burden level gets too high.

YOUR BODY'S ABILITY TO DETOXIFY

Your body uses 5 main organs to detoxify from environmental and internal toxins—your liver, kidneys, colon, lungs, and skin. The lymphatic system can also be included because of its role in waste removal and fighting invaders such as bacteria and viruses.

These organs and their related systems maintain the health of your body by transforming and/or eliminating the foreign substances that you are exposed to.

FAT SOLUBLE TOXINS

One major problem is that some toxins are fat soluble and therefore are unable to be fully eliminated by the body. Instead, these fat soluble toxins are stored in the lipid membrane of each cell and your body's actual fat cells. Studies confirm that everyone, including children, have various toxic compounds stored in their fatty (adipose) tissue.[2]

Studies confirm that everyone, including children, have various toxic compounds stored in their fat tissue.

DETOXIFYING YOUR BODY

Your body's ability to metabolize and eliminate toxins can be enhanced by improving the function of the organs responsible for detoxification and elimination. This can result in more energy, better sleep, elevated mood, and a reduction of many common health problems.

This leads to the **third body essential of health and wellness —*detoxification*.**

By following the recommendations outlined later in this chapter, you will assist your body to detoxify from both environmental and internal toxins. As your toxic burden level is reduced, your overall state of health will improve—physically, mentally, and emotionally.

Before these natural detoxification methods are considered, it is crucial to first reduce or eliminate the root causes of toxicity.

REDUCING YOUR EXPOSURE

The following section outlines some of the most impactful factors that contribute to your body's toxic burden level along with methods to reduce or eliminate your exposure to them.

SOURCES OF TOXINS

YOUR DIET

In Chapter 2 you learned that one way to decrease your intake of toxins is by eating quality organic food, as it reduces the amount of pesticides and drug residues you ingest.[7,8] Quality organic foods also tend to contain less preservatives, additives, and colorings than conventional foods.

By following the diet recommendations in Chapter 2, you support the detoxification pathways (especially your liver, colon, and kidneys) by providing these organs with the essential vitamins, minerals, essential fatty acids, fiber, and other nutrients required for effective detoxification. Without these nutrients, your body's ability to process and eliminate toxins is compromised.

> *By following the diet recommendations in Chapter 2 you support the detoxification pathways.*

When cooking, use stainless steel, ceramic, and glass. Non-stick coatings on cookware have been shown to release toxic fumes when used at temperatures over 350° Celsius (650° Fahrenheit).[1]

The water you drink can also be a source of toxins—chlorine being the main one. Chlorine does kill pathogens in our water but is a chemical toxin.[9] If possible, use a high quality water filter in your home. One company that supplies water filtration systems specifically for water in Vancouver, B.C. can be found at www.yourwatermatters.com.

Bottled water in plastic containers may be convenient, but some studies reveal that it may not be all that pristine. Bacteria, toxic metals, and chemicals such as BPA and plasticizers have been found in samples.[10] The healthiest, most environmentally friendly, and most economical solution is to filter your own and use stainless steel or glass water bottles.

HOUSEHOLD AND BODY CLEANSERS

Standard cleaning products that you use on your body and in your home often contain a myriad of chemicals. Explore using more natural based products that are free of harsh chemicals. Most health food stores and some grocery stores carry natural alternatives. Also, remember what goes down your drain goes into the ecosystem of the planet and eventually recycles back into you.

ENVIRONMENTAL POLLUTION

One recent study tested the blood of 11 individuals across Canada for 88 different toxic chemicals.[3] On average 44 toxic chemicals were found in the participants blood including fire retardants, stain repellants, pesticides, mercury, lead, DDT, and PCBs.

The chemicals detected are known to cause reproductive disorders, harm the development of children, disrupt the hormonal system, and are suspected of causing cancer and respiratory illness.

As environmental laws improve and industries move toward

"greener" production methods, exposure to toxic chemicals in the environment will hopefully decline.

Until that happens, make wise choices and avoid possible sources of exposure. You can also minimize your contribution to environmental toxins by implementing the "reduce, reuse, and recycle" philosophy.

For more in depth information on environmental pollution and your health, visit www.slowdeathbyrubberduck.com.

One study found an average of 44 toxic chemicals in the blood of individuals tested from across Canada.

MERCURY DENTAL FILLINGS

Mercury is a heavy metal and powerful neurotoxin that is capable of creating neurological, psychological, and immunological changes.[11] Studies have shown that mercury dental fillings leach toxic mercury into the body.[12,13] More and more dentists are moving away from using mercury fillings and some specialize in their safe removal.

Sweden, Denmark, and Norway have banned the use of mercury in dental fillings, and other countries are beginning to implement severe restrictions.

Recently, the FDA in the United States made a statement on their website: "Dental amalgams contain mercury, which may have neurotoxic effects on the nervous systems of developing children and fetuses."[14]

Health Canada states on their website: "As a general principle, it is advisable to reduce human exposure to heavy metals in our environment, even if there is no clinical evidence of adverse health effects, provided the reduction can be achieved at reasonable cost and without introducing other adverse effects."[13]

If you have mercury fillings, consider having them replaced with another material by a dentist who specializes in safe removal.

For more information on the effects of mercury amalgam fillings, and for referrals to biological dentists trained in the safe removal of mercury amalgams, visit the website of the International Academy of Oral Medicine and Toxicology at www.iaomt.org.

> *Recently, the FDA in the United States stated that mercury fillings can cause health problems in children and fetuses.*

VACCINATIONS

After decades of use, vaccine manufacturers have finally removed thimerosal (the mercury derived preservative) from most vaccines. (According to an article in the Los Angeles Times on Feb 8, 2005, vaccine manufacturer Merck knew as early as 1991 that children following the recommended vaccine schedule were receiving 87 times the amount of mercury considered safe.) Currently in Canada, mercury is still present in some vaccines such as the flu shot and in some hepatitis B shots.

Most vaccines still contain aluminum, formaldehyde, and other preservatives.[15] Aluminum, like mercury, is also a neurotoxin and accumulates in the body's tissues. A recent study on the effects of aluminum hydroxide (the aluminum used in vaccines) showed significant neurological damage in mice.[16]

Many people, including parents and some physicians, have concerns over the safety of vaccines and their potential short and long term side effects. Part of this concern is due to the dramatic increase in the number of vaccines in the current recommended childhood vaccination schedule.

In 1983, the Centers for Disease Control (CDC) recommended children get 10 vaccine shots for 7 different diseases by the age of 6. Today that number has climbed to 36 shots for 14 different diseases by the age of 6—an increase of 260 percent.[17]

As vaccine manufacturers produce more vaccines for children, the importance of making an educated decision on how, when, and whether or not to vaccinate becomes increasingly important.

Some medical doctors recommend an alternative to the government recommended vaccine schedule. Refer to the references in this footnote for more information.[18,19]

If you or your child are getting vaccinated, avoid ones that contain mercury. Also, maintain contact with your natural health care professional for adjunctive supportive measures.

Most vaccines still contain aluminum, formaldehyde, and other preservatives.

ELECTROMAGNETIC RADIATION

Electromagnetic radiation comes from exposure to power lines and radiation from all electrical devices such as computers, wireless routers, cordless phones, cell phone towers, and most importantly—cell phones.

Research has revealed that the electromagnetic radiation from cell phones has detrimental biological effects on the body. Studies have linked cell phone use to brain tumors and an impairment of male fertility.[20,21]

Frequent exposure to cell phone radiation has also become a serious concern for younger children (including the fetuses of pregnant women) whose brains and skulls are still developing.

In July 2008, the Toronto Department of Public Health announced a warning on cell phone use in children stating: "Today's children have started to use cell phones at a younger age, therefore their lifetime exposure to cell phone RFs (radiofrequencies) will likely be greater. As a result, the chances that a child could develop harmful health effects from using a cell phone for a long time may be greater."[22]

Cell phone use in prenatal and postnatal women has also been linked to behavior problems such as hyperactivity and emotional problems in their children.[23]

Use your cell phone as little as possible. If you do need to use it, use a speaker phone or a specific headset designed to reduce radiation exposure. If you are carrying your cell phone close to your body, keep it turned off until you need to use it. Young children should not use cell phones except in emergency situations.

If you have a wireless router in your home, consider going back to a cabled version. At the very least, shut it off at night or when not in use. Recently the German government advised its citizens to avoid using wireless connections as a way to reduce personal exposure to "electrosmog".

Before more research is conducted in this area, it's best to err on the side caution by taking steps to reduce exposure to electromagnetic radiation.

> *Research has revealed that the electromagnetic radiation from cell phones has detrimental biological effects on the body.*

THE MEDIA

Although not typically thought of as a type of contamination, today's media exposure could easily been seen as a type of mental pollution. Everywhere we go we are inundated with information and advertisements. Television, newspapers, magazines, billboards, and of course the internet—all attempt to tell us what is important and what is deemed to be "news".

While it is good to be informed, you might find it helpful to reduce or eliminate your intake of unnecessary and negative information. Try taking a break from these influences for a period of time and observe how you feel.

NATURAL METHODS OF DETOXIFICATION

This next section introduces three essential and effective methods that you can use to help detoxify your body. You may choose to do one of the detoxification methods or all three. Each one has a specific effect and benefit.

1. Cardiovascular Exercise

2. Sauna Therapy

3. Dietary Cleanse

There are recommendations at the end of this chapter on how to select which method is best for you at this time.

DETOXIFICATION ESSENTIAL #1: CARDIOVASCULAR EXERCISE

Exercise is a crucial ingredient to enhance your body's detoxifying abilities. From reading Chapter 1, you know that exercise can improve the function of every bodily system. This includes your organs of detoxification and elimination—your lungs, liver, kidneys, colon, and skin.

Cardiovascular exercise in particular, strongly stimulates circulation, metabolism, oxygenation, perspiration, and lymph flow—all essential components for whole body health.

Human and animal studies have also shown that endurance exercise training develops the body's ability to maintain higher levels of glutathione in the liver and other tissues of the body.[24,25] Glutathione protects against oxidative damage and is necessary for cellular and liver detoxification.

Cardiovascular exercise (running, biking, swimming, aerobics, etc.) strongly increases respiration. Deep diaphragmatic breathing pumps the diaphragm and rib cage, creating a massage like action on organs such as the lungs, liver, and intestines improving the function of these organs.

Cardiovascular exercise also increases metabolism and perspiration—both of which can assist the body to mobilize and release toxins stored in the body's fat cells.

> *Cardiovascular exercise is an essential method of enhancing your body's detoxifying abilities.*

THE 3 WEEK CARDIO DETOX

1. Engage in a cardiovascular activity that increases respiration and perspiration for at least 15 minutes three times per week for 3 consistent weeks. Refer to Chapter 1 for exercise ideas.

2. You can combine your cardio detox with your action plan from Chapter 1 by doing your cardiovascular exercise on your challenge days.

3. At the end of the 3 weeks, maintain your results by continuing with at least 1 day per week of cardiovascular exercise.

4. Follow the supplement protocol and dietary recommendations outlined below.

THE 3 WEEK CARDIO DETOX SUPPLEMENT PROTOCOL

The following supplements are suggested to support your body while doing The 3 Week Cardio Detox. They specifically support the adrenal glands which are often taxed and exhausted in many people due to stress. By supporting and nourishing your adrenal glands, you will have the energy needed to exercise.

These supplements are suggested in addition to The Top 3 Supplements listed in Chapter 2. In addition to all the benefits mentioned in Chapter 2 on fish oils, the omega 3 fatty acids contained in fish reduce inflammation in the body and are also capable of reducing the effects of stress on the adrenal glands.[26] During The 3 Week Cardio Detox be sure to take your fish oil supplement daily. (Vegetarians can substitute fresh walnut, flaxseed and flax oil, although they are less potent than fish oils.)

B-VITAMIN SUPPLEMENT

B-vitamins counteract stress, promote a healthy nervous system, and are required for energy production. Vitamin B5 in particular is found in high amounts in the adrenal glands. Supplement your diet with a high quality multi B-vitamin (1–2 per day).

VITAMIN C

Like vitamin B5, vitamin C is also found in high amounts in the adrenal glands. Both of these vitamins are water soluble and can be used up quickly, especially during periods of stress. Take 500mg once or twice daily, with meals. *Cold types* as described at the end of this chapter should take the lower dosage as vitamin C has a cooling effect on the body. *Hot types* will find the upper dosage most beneficial.

SIBERIAN GINSENG *(ELEUTHEROCOCCUS SENTICOSUS)*

This herb is known to counteract stress and fatigue and increase physical endurance and concentration. It also has anti-inflammatory and anti-arthritic properties and bolsters immunity. Take 60–90 drops of the tincture two to three times per day, or 1000mg – 1500mg of the herb in capsule form two to three times per day. Follow the directions on the bottle for concentrated extracts. (This herb should not be taken during acute inflammations or colds and flus.)

At the end of the 3 weeks, gradually reduce dosage of supplements over a few days and then only take as needed. Integrate some of the following superfoods into your diet for long term health.

THE 3 WEEK CARDIO DETOX DIETARY RECOMMENDATIONS

Be sure to include a serving of protein and healthy fats with each meal to stabilize blood sugar levels (see Chapter 2: *Fats and Oils*), and implement at least *The Top 6 Essentials* from Chapter 2. If you drink coffee, switch to organic green tea as coffee taxes the adrenal glands. Green tea does contain caffeine, but much less than coffee or black tea, and is also beneficial to the liver. Licorice tea is also recommended during this program as licorice herb is very beneficial for the adrenal glands. Drink one or two cups per day. (Licorice is not advised for those with high blood pressure.)

SUPERFOODS

As an alternative to supplements, include these "superfoods" into your regular diet. These foods not only have superb nutritional profiles, but they also have specific effects upon the energetics of the body as defined by traditional Chinese medicine.

Here are the definitions of some terms used to describe the benefits of these foods:

Chi	The vital life energy of the body.
Yin	The cooling, nourishing, fluid aspects of the body.
Yang	The warmth and strength of the body. Yang moves the circulation and warms the digestion.
Kidneys	The house of the vital essence of health and wellness. The kidneys also include the adrenal glands.
Blood	The blood and its ability to moisten and nourish the body.

THE FOODS

◊ walnuts (high in omega 3 fats, tonifies kidney yang)

◊ flax seeds (omega 3 fats)

◊ black sesame seeds (high calcium, tonifies kidney yin)

◊ blackstrap molasses (high minerals such as iron and calcium, B-vitamins, tonifies blood)

◊ butter from grass fed cows (omega 3 fats and saturated fat)

◊ wild salmon (high omega 3 fats)

◊ unrefined sea salt (essential minerals)

◊ goji berries, blueberries, dark grapes, black currants, raspberries, and blackberries (antioxidants, tonifies blood, yin, and chi)

◊ black beans (high antioxidant, B-vitamins, tonifies kidneys)

◊ seaweeds such as dulse, kombu, and kelp (high minerals)

◊ garlic (strengthens digestion, detoxifies, tonifies yang)

REVISITING YOUR HEALTH ACCOUNT

During The 3 Week Cardio Detox, you may notice an appreciable increase in your energy and vitality. How you use this energy is up to you. You may either spend it on lifestyle habits that have a depleting effect on your health account (late nights, high stress, overworking, overeating unhealthy food, etc.), or you may choose to bank this vitality into your health account.

In traditional Chinese medicine, two types of vital life energy, or "chi", are described. One is called "ancestral chi" and the other "acquired chi". Ancestral chi is the energy that you inherit when you are born. This energy can only be spent during your life—not increased. On the other hand, acquired chi can be increased and stored. The most important ways to do this are through healthy diet, proper breathing and exercise, and meditative practices. The more acquired chi that we develop, the less we have to tap into our ancestral chi. Ancestral and acquired chi are like health dollars in your health account, as described in Chapter 1.

DETOXIFICATION ESSENTIAL #2: SAUNA THERAPY

Using heat to induce sweating is another way of stimulating the skin's ability to eliminate. For hundreds of years, cultures throughout the world such as the Finnish, Russians, Native Americans, and Japanese have used sweat therapy as a means of improving physical, mental, emotional, and spiritual wellness.

In recent years, sauna therapy has drawn attention as a means of detoxifying the body from toxic metals and other substances that are stored in the body.

One study showed a reduction of concentration levels of hexachlorobenzene, pesticides, and polychlorinated biphenyl congeners (PCBs) in adipose (fat) tissue, following a program of sauna use, exercise, and dietary supplementation.[27]

Other studies have shown the presence of toxic metals such as lead, cadmium, and mercury in sweat.[28-30] Medications and other drugs are also readily detectable in sweat.[31,32]

Although the science behind sauna therapy is still emerging, it is thought that repeated sauna sessions can detoxify the whole body. Heat increases metabolism, circulation, and fluid exchange in the body—potentially allowing toxins to be mobilized from the body's connective tissues, fat cells, and cell membranes. These toxins are then excreted through the skin during perspiration, or metabolized and eliminated through the liver, colon, lungs, and kidneys.

More research needs to be done, but many doctors have reported improved health in their patients who have used sauna therapy.

Sauna therapy helps the body mobilize and eliminate stored toxins.

OTHER BENEFITS OF SAUNA

During a sauna, circulation of the whole body increases dramatically. Blood vessels dilate, muscles and tendons loosen and relax, and fluid exchange increases through perspiration and lymphatic flow.

People diagnosed with chronic pain or fibromyalgia often find sauna use beneficial.

Acupuncturists and energy workers understand that where tension exists, there will be corresponding blockages in the flow of energy or "chi". Since sauna therapy releases tension and improves circulation, energy flow can also be improved. Blocked energy creates pain and disease, while free flowing energy creates health and wellness.

Sauna therapy is also beneficial during the initial stages of colds and flus as it stimulates the immune system, and results in faster healing response.[33] Moderate fevers should not be stifled because they help the body fight the infecting virus.

Periodic saunas for relaxation and cleansing the skin can also be enjoyed.

PRECAUTIONS FOR SAUNA THERAPY

If you are taking prescribed medication or have any health concerns like heart disease, high blood pressure, diabetes or epilepsy, or have metal parts in your body, you should consult with your physician before using a sauna. Do not use a sauna if you are pregnant or breastfeeding, have an acute injury, enclosed infection, predisposition to hemorrhaging, or are on prescription steroids.

SAUNA THERAPY FOR MOTHERS-TO-BE

A detoxification protocol that includes sauna therapy is highly recommended for women who are intending to get pregnant. Lowering your body's toxic burden level will reduce the amount of toxins that are passed on to your infant through your breast milk and umbilical blood.

Start preparing your body for pregnancy by implementing sauna therapy routines up to one year before planning to conceive. Stop sauna therapy 2–3 months prior to conception to give your body a chance to focus on building reserves—rather than on eliminating.

THE BENEFITS OF CHLORELLA

Chlorella is a micro-algae that has the ability to bind to toxic metals and environmental toxins in the digestive tract and carry them out through the stool.

In one study, pregnant women supplemented with chlorella for a period of approximately 6 months. The results showed a decrease in dioxin (an environmental toxin) levels and an increase in immunoglobulin A (IgA—a part of the immune system) in breast milk.[34] Increased breast milk IgA levels may benefit nursing infants by reducing the risk of infections.

Chlorella is also a superfood that is high in vitamins such as B12 and B6, chlorophyll, minerals, protein, beta-carotene, and fatty acids. It can be found in most health food stores. Choose brands with a "cracked cell wall".

INFRARED SAUNAS

Infrared saunas use infrared light to penetrate and heat the body from the inside to create perspiration, whereas traditional saunas heat the surrounding air which then heats the body. As a result infrared saunas typically operate at lower temperatures than traditional saunas, allowing for a more comfortable option.

Infrared saunas are also thought to be more effective for detoxification due to the penetrating effect of infrared rays on the body.

Some health centres, tanning salons, and other businesses offer infrared sauna use as a service. Easy to assemble small units can be purchased making sauna therapy instantly available in your own home.

THE 4 WEEK SAUNA DETOX

This can be done once or twice per year—spring and fall.

1. Do 3 sauna sessions per week for a period of 4 weeks.

2. Start with one heating session of 5–10 minutes. If this is comfortable, increase to 15–20 minutes. You should be sweating profusely by this point. Time frames may need to be adjusted depending on temperature and the type of sauna used.

3. If comfortable, build up to 3 intervals of 15–20 minutes each, with a 5–10 minute rest/cool down period between heating sessions. Leave the sauna and sit or lie down.

4. Follow the supplement protocol outlined below.

THE 4 WEEK SAUNA DETOX SUPPLEMENT PROTOCOL

The following herbs and supplements should be used during The 4 Week Sauna Detox to support your detoxification pathways and encourage the elimination of toxins. These products can be found in most health food stores and are suggested in addition to The Top 3 Supplements listed in Chapter 2. Because sauna therapy increases your body's usage and demand for many nutrients such as magnesium, increase the dosage of your multivitamin to the highest recommended dosage. (Some brands allow up to 6 capsules per day.) If your multivitamin does not contain calcium and magnesium, or does not contain at least 250mg of magnesium at maximum dosage, add a calcium/magnesium supplement to your daily regime during the sauna detox. Take your fish oil and probiotic supplements daily.

It is crucial that you are supporting your body with wise food choices by following the diet recommendations in Chapter 2. Be sure to boost your daily intake of green leafy veggies. Also, make sure you are doing your regular days and challenge days from Chapter 1. Your body needs movement to heal, stay healthy, and detoxify.

CILANTRO TINCTURE *(CORIANDRUM SATIVUM)*

Studies have shown that cilantro has the ability to mobilize and detoxify heavy metals such as lead and mercury.[35,36] As your body eliminates toxins during the sauna detox, cilantro can be used to help mobilize and eliminate stored toxins. For this purpose, take 10 drops of the tincture twice per day on sauna days.

MILK THISTLE *(SILYBUM MARIANUM)*

Milk thistle is an herb that helps protect the liver from toxins.[37] It has been extensively studied and shown to be effective against many toxic substances including the highly potent liver toxin from the death cap mushroom (*amanita phalloides*).

During sauna therapy some of the toxins that become mobilized will be processed by the liver. To protect it during this process, take 200mg of milk thistle extract (in capsule form) twice daily with meals.

GARLIC

Garlic is abundant in sulphur and selenium—both needed for detoxification. Fresh garlic holds strong antimicrobial properties for killing off yeast, bacteria, and other organisms in the digestive tract.[38-40] Take 1 clove of chopped fresh garlic once per day before meals 3–5 days per week. Take with water—don't chew. If fresh garlic isn't tolerated, cooked garlic or garlic capsules may be substituted as they are still high in sulphur and selenium.

A FEW TIPS TO USING A SAUNA

BEFORE USING A SAUNA

◊ Make sure you are well hydrated before, during, and after your sauna.

◊ Don't eat a heavy meal or have an empty stomach just before using a sauna. Eat lightly before going in and a little afterwards if needed. A piece of fruit may suffice.

◊ Optional: Do 5–20 minutes of cardiovascular exercise before entering the sauna to open up deeper levels of circulation and to further stimulate metabolism.

◊ 110–130° Fahrenheit is usually appropriate for most people using an infrared sauna.

◊ Sauna with a buddy for safety.

WHILE IN THE SAUNA

◊ If at any time you experience headache, dizziness, cramps, irregular heartbeat or shortness of breath—leave the sauna immediately.

◊ Wipe off the sweat as you perspire to encourage more sweating and to clear any toxic residues.

◊ Drink water mixed with fresh juice and a few pinches of sea salt to maintain electrolyte levels in your body, especially if you are doing more than one heating session.

◊ Massage the acupressure points in Figs. 1–3 during each round in the sauna to support the detoxification process.

AFTER SAUNA

◊ A short cool shower immediately after using the sauna can be used to stimulate circulation throughout the whole body. It's an invigorating must to complete the sauna experience! (Not advised for those with heart conditions.) Begin immersing one limb at a time, starting furthest from the heart—right leg, left leg, right arm, left arm, then the rest of the body and head. Rinse off—don't use soap.

◊ Take a light 5–10 minute walk after using the sauna to move your muscles and joints and to get some fresh air. Breathe deeply.

◊ Make sure you are having regular bowel movements while undergoing sauna therapy to ensure healthy elimination.

Be sure to read *The Detoxification Process* section at the end of this chapter for additional recommendations.

ACUPRESSURE POINTS FOR SAUNA THERAPY

Once you warm up in the sauna, massage these three acupressure points firmly on both sides of your body for 60 seconds each. Massaging them will help your body adjust to the heat and detoxification process. They are specifically important points for the liver, kidneys, large intestine, and immune system.

KIDNEY (FIG.1)

During a sauna, heat (yang) tends to rise in the body and dry up the cooling, fluid aspect of the body (yin). This point helps to descend hot energy by stimulating the kidney chi. It also helps to prevent headaches, dizziness, and other effects of heat such as ringing in the ears, hot flashes, anger, high blood pressure, and palpitations.

First Aid Tip: Pressing very firmly on this point as well as a point located in the middle of the space between the upper lip and the nose can help revive someone who has passed out.

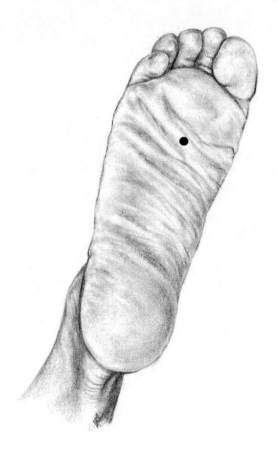

LIVER (FIG.2)

The liver has an aversion to heat, so it's important to help keep it cool by massaging this point. Also, as toxins are mobilized in the body the liver can become congested as it processes them. Massaging this point will help the liver detoxify more effectively by clearing any excess heat in it. It also helps to avert headaches by preventing heat (yang) from rising in the body.

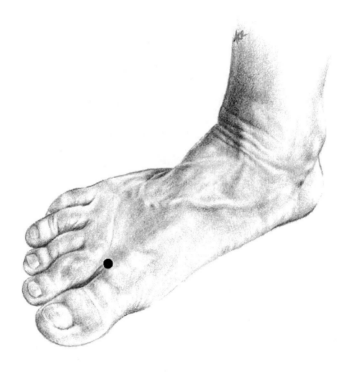

LARGE INTESTINE (FIG.3)

This important point helps the body adjust to the sweating process and release pathogenic energy (known as "wind" in Chinese medicine) through the skin. It can relieve pain anywhere in the body and is especially helpful for relieving headaches. It also clears stagnant energy, strengthens chi and immunity, and can be useful in treating colds and flus. It should not be used by pregnant women. Press into the middle of the web between the thumb and forefinger with pressure directed towards the bone of the forefinger.

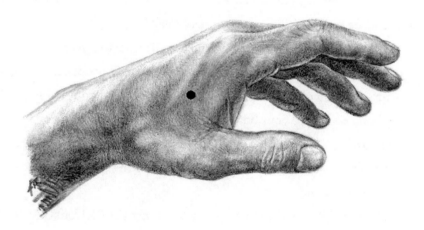

DETOXIFICATION ESSENTIAL #3: DIETARY CLEANSES

Dietary cleanses are another way to help your body detoxify. There are many types of dietary cleanses. Some involve the complete abstinence of food by fasting, while more moderate approaches eliminate specific foods and calories.

Reducing and simplifying your food intake for a period of time gives your digestive system a well deserved rest from working its usual 24/7. Digestion is optimized and the organs of detoxification function more efficiently. This process allows your body to "digest" the physical, mental, and emotional excesses it has been carrying—resulting in the emergence of a more balanced state of health.

Dietary cleanses can also focus on eliminating yeast, bacteria or parasites in the body improving digestion and absorption. These critters are also capable of releasing their own toxic compounds into your body adding to your body's toxic burden level. Specific foods and herbs can be used in a dietary cleanse to target these microbes and to improve the health of your detoxification organs such as the bowel, liver, and kidneys.

Doing a dietary cleanse also gives your body a break from the ingestion of possible food sensitivities, food additives, processed foods, sugars, unhealthy fats, and other unhealthy foods—allowing it to return to a state of balance.

Once or twice a year is recommended—preferably in the spring or fall when your body is adjusting from the extremes of summer and winter.

CLEANSING BODY, MIND, AND SPIRIT

Dietary cleanses aren't limited to a physical experience of the body—they also serve to heal the mind and spirit. As you dramatically shift one aspect of your life, all other areas are affected.

Fasting or cleansing can be a time to re-evaluate your life and create a foundation for change. It is advised to slow down, reduce your activities, and become more introspective during a dietary cleanse.

Like sweat therapy, many cultures have used dietary cleanses for hundreds of years to purify body, mind, and spirit.

> *Dietary cleanses aren't limited to a physical experience of the body. They also serve to heal the mind and spirit.*

START WITH A HEALTHY FOUNDATION

Proper long term eating and lifestyle habits provide the best health insurance, but a good dietary cleanse consisting of mostly nutrient dense, fiber rich vegetables, can give your system a boost of vitality.

If you are just starting to make positive changes in your lifestyle, I suggest you implement the recommended changes from Chapter 1 and 2 for two weeks before embarking on The 3 Day Cleanse. These changes begin the detoxification process and prepare your body with a foundation for deeper cleansing.

Do not do a dietary cleanse if you are underweight, malnourished, or pregnant. In these cases, emphasis should be on building the body's strength and reserves through good nutrition and other therapeutic measures.

THE 3 DAY CLEANSE

The 3 Day Cleanse is a simple dietary cleanse designed to detoxify the whole body as well as eliminate yeast, fungi, parasites, and harmful bacteria from the digestive tract.

As your microbial load is reduced, stress is removed from the liver as it no longer has to metabolize toxins released from the microbes. Digestion and absorption in the small intestine is improved, and your immune system strengthened.[41]

Exercises for body, mind, and spirit are included in The 3 Day Cleanse to assist with the holistic process of cleansing.

It is important to note that stresses and habitual mental/emotional patterns cause toxins to be held in the body tissues. This point was made during a lecture by Dr. Klinghardt, MD, PhD. He described a case of a woman he was treating using intravenous chelation who released incredibly high amounts of mercury in her urine immediately after resolving a mental/emotional conflict. Prior to this resolution, very little mercury was being released indicating that her mental/emotional state was causing her body to retain the mercury.

By resolving unhealthy beliefs and negative emotions, a deeper level of detoxification occurs resulting in a transformation of body, mind, and spirit—the real purpose for doing a dietary cleanse.

THE 3 DAY CLEANSE

For 3 consecutive days, do the following:

UPON ARISING

Start each day by steeping 2–3 slices of fresh raw ginger in hot water to make tea. Add the juice from a thin slice of freshly squeezed lemon, and a half teaspoon of honey.

BEFORE EACH MEAL (3 TIMES PER DAY)

Take 60–90 drops of dandelion root tincture.

BREAKFAST

Cooked brown rice with steamed green leafy vegetables and at least one other steamed or baked veggie (see suggested list) with a little flax oil or unrefined organic olive oil.

LUNCH

Cooked lentils with steamed green leafy vegetables and at least one other steamed or baked veggie (see suggested list) with a little flax oil or unrefined organic olive oil. If doing your cleanse in hot weather, a serving of raw vegetables may be included.

AFTERNOON SNACK

1 piece of fresh locally grown in season fruit.

DINNER

15 minutes before meal, chop 1 clove of fresh garlic and take with water—don't chew.

Black beans with steamed green leafy vegetables and at least one other steamed or baked veggie (see suggested list) with a little flax oil or unrefined organic olive oil, plus a serving of unpasteurized sauerkraut. A small serving of raw veggies is permitted year round.

GINGER TEA WITH LEMON AND HONEY

Ginger increases circulation and movement, lemon juice helps cleanse the digestive tract, and honey lubricates the colon.[42] This tea is also excellent for treating colds and flus.

BROWN RICE

Brown rice is a nutrient dense food that is gluten-free and generally hypoallergenic. It contains high levels of manganese, selenium, and magnesium, and also contains B-vitamins, vitamin E, fiber, fatty acids, iron, and a spectrum of phytonutrients. Refined polished white rice is stripped of nearly all these nutrients. Choose organic brown rice if possible and store the dry grain in the refrigerator to protect its oils. Leftovers should also be stored in the refrigerator in a tightly sealed container to preserve freshness.

Keep cooked serving size to ½ to ¾ cup.

To Prepare Brown Rice:

Rinse first. Add ¾ cup of brown rice to 1½ cups of water. Cover and bring to a boil. Simmer for 45 minutes or until soft.

Makes 3–4 servings.

LENTILS

Lentils are one of the easiest beans to digest and provide an excellent vegetarian protein source during the cleanse. Protein helps to stabilize blood sugar levels. A simple meal of lentils and vegetables—without the carbohydrates from grains—digests well in most people.[43] Complete digestion is required to avoid the overgrowth of microbes such as yeast and bacteria in the digestive tract.[43] Below is a simple recipe for cooking lentils (Indian dahl).

Keep cooked serving sizes to ½ to ¾ cup.

To prepare:

Rinse and soak ½ cup of lentils in 2 cups of water overnight. Sort out any stones first. Discard water after soaking.

Put the soaked lentils in a pot with 1¼ cups of fresh water and bring to a boil. Then cover and simmer for 30–60 minutes or until tender. (Some types cook faster.) Optional: place a strip of kombu seaweed in the bottom of the pot before cooking for added nutrients and easier digestion.

Near end of cooking add:

- ¼ teaspoon sea salt
- ¼ teaspoon ground cumin
- ¼ teaspoon ground coriander
- ¼ teaspoon turmeric

Cumin, coriander, and turmeric assist digestion and reduce gas. Turmeric is also good for the liver and holds anti-inflammatory properties.[44] All these spices are warming to the digestive system.

Makes 2–3 servings.

STEAMED GREEN LEAFY VEGGIES

Broccoli, cabbage, watercress, Swiss chard, kale, and collards are good choices. Other than Swiss chard, all belong to the cruciferous family which holds detoxifying properties for the liver.[45] Eat as many of them as you like. A little flax oil or unrefined organic olive oil can be drizzled on them.

OTHER VEGETABLES OF YOUR CHOICE

In addition to your serving of green leafy vegetables, choose at least one more fresh vegetable to steam or bake other than potatoes as they are high in starch, and avoid corn, tomatoes, sweet peppers, and egg plant as these are common food sensitivities. Artichokes, asparagus, beets, zucchini, onions, turnips, pumpkin, squash, yams, sweet potatoes, and carrots are a few possibilities. Artichoke is especially beneficial to the liver and gall bladder.[46]

BLACK BEANS

Like lentils, black beans are high in protein, fiber, B-vitamins, iron, and trace minerals such as manganese. Black beans are also a superfood—they are very high in antioxidants and traditional Chinese medicine considers them a nutritive tonic to the kidney/adrenal glands. Because the quality of canned beans is close to that of dried beans, you may use canned organic black beans (Yves® brand recommended) unless you are familiar with cooking your own. Simply heat them on the stove and eat plain or add some chopped fresh cilantro or a pinch of the spices used for the lentils. Keep cooked serving size to ½ to ¾ cup. Black beans are heavier to digest than lentils, so if you are not used to eating beans—or have difficulty digesting them—substitute black beans for lentils from the lunch menu. See *"Other Dietary Suggestions"* for more recommendations on improving digestion.

UNPASTEURIZED SAUERKRAUT

Unpasteurized sauerkraut contains healthy active bacterial cultures that are beneficial for digestion. These bacteria are killed off in the process of pasteurization therefore the sauerkraut you buy must be unpasteurized. It can be purchased in some health food stores. Eat as much as you like.

If unpasteurized sauerkraut is not available, take a probiotic supplement containing the healthy bacteria strains *L. acidophilus* and *bifidobacterium*. This supplement is used to boost friendly bacteria in the gut. Take 1–2 capsules once per day with food. Yogurt is not permitted.

After finishing the cleanse, continue to implement fermented foods into your diet such as unpasteurized sauerkraut, kefir, unpasteurized miso, and quality yogurt.

ONE PIECE OF FRUIT

Choose local, fresh, and in season fruit if available. Avoid tropical fruit unless you live in the tropics. If you are doing the cleanse in the summer, an extra serving of fruit per day is allowed. If you are doing it in the winter, only one serving of cooked fruit is permitted such as homemade applesauce, blueberries warmed up on the stove, etc. Add a little cinnamon, nutmeg, or cardamom to cooked fruit to add a warming energy and to aid digestion.

FRESH GARLIC

Fresh raw garlic has strong antimicrobial properties.[38-40] It kills yeast, bacteria, parasites, and fungi in the digestive tract. Once garlic is cooked or processed (capsules) it loses much of this property. Garlic is also high in sulphur and selenium—both helpful for detoxifying mercury and other heavy metals from the body. If fresh garlic isn't tolerated or for those with *hot* constitutions, oregano oil may be preferred. (See *Selecting a Detoxification Method* on pages 103 and 104 for a description of the hot and cold constitutions.) Oregano oil also holds antimicrobial properties. It is also good for colds that begin in the throat. It can be found in most health food stores. Take 3–5 drops twice daily, between meals.

At the end of the 3 days, continue taking the garlic or oregano oil for a few more days as you integrate back into a normal diet.

> **Traveler's Tip:** The antimicrobial action of fresh garlic and oregano oil makes them both useful for minor digestive issues associated with consuming food of questionable hygiene. Like probiotic supplements, they are valuable to have on hand when travelling to some areas.

DANDELION ROOT TINCTURE

This high-mineral herb helps detoxify the liver, is a diuretic, and also acts as a mild laxative to ensure the bowels keep moving properly while on the cleanse.[47] The tincture can be found in most health food stores. (Capsules may be substituted for tincture for those who want to avoid alcohol.) Do not use this herb if you have gall bladder inflammation or bile duct obstruction, and use with caution if you have gallstones.

At the end of the 3 days, continue taking the dandelion tincture at half dosage for a few more days as you integrate back into a normal diet.

OTHER DIETARY SUGGESTIONS

◊ Only eat the foods listed in the menu. Continue any prescribed medications, but stop taking any additional supplements.

◊ Organic foods are best. Choose whenever possible.

◊ Eat as many vegetables as you like but every meal must include a green leafy one.

◊ Fennel tea is recommended for reducing gas and improving digestion—drink a cup after lunch and dinner. Water and other herbal teas such as chamomile, ginger, rooibos, holy basil, and peppermint are permitted and can also be helpful. Because green tea contains caffeine, avoid it during the cleanse. No sweeteners, milk or juices.

◊ For added flavor and improved digestion, use herbs such as basil, oregano, rosemary, thyme, and sage to season your veggies. These are especially beneficial at breakfast and for those with a cold constitution. No hot spices or black pepper, no sauces or dressings, and no salt other than what is added to the lentils. (Canned black beans usually have salt added.)

◊ Fresh parsley and cilantro can be eaten with meals as desired. Parsley is high in vitamins and minerals, supports the kidneys, acts as a diuretic, and assists digestion.[48] Cilantro has the ability to detoxify heavy metals.[35,36]

◊ If unpasteurized sauerkraut is not available, take a teaspoon of organic raw apple cider vinegar in a bit of water before dinner to aid digestion and acidify the gut. This helps counteract microbes such as bacteria and yeast.

COMPLIMENTARY PRACTICES

MOVEMENT

During The 3 Day Cleanse, walk daily for at least 15 minutes outside or do any other regular day activity from Chapter 1, but do not do any challenge days. Cleansing is a time to turn inwards and reflect. In Chinese medicine it would be considered a *yin* time. Challenge days are more *yang*—expressive and intense. Be gentle and quiet in mind and body for the 3 days.

MEDITATIVE PRACTICE

Each day of The 3 Day Cleanse, practice *The 3 Step Self-Healing Protocol* as taught in *Book 3: Spirit*, and if desired, any of the exercises taught in *Book 2: Mind*. Alternatively, you could use any other type of meditation, prayer, or relaxation practice that you might be familiar with.

INTROSPECTION

In *Book 3: Spirit*, you will learn how gratitude has the power to change your mind and body and how it connects you to your true Self. Take a few minutes at the end of each day to ask yourself: "What am I grateful for today?" Share your answer with a family member or friend, or write it down in a journal.

SHOPPING LIST FOR THE 3 DAY CLEANSE

◊ lentils (about 1 cup or 2 cups if substituting lentils for black beans)

◊ organic canned black beans (2 cans, Yves® brand recommended)

◊ green leafy vegetables (9 meals)

◊ other vegetables (9 meals)

◊ local fruit (3–6 servings, depending on season)

◊ brown rice (about 1 cup dried)

◊ flax oil or organic unrefined olive oil

◊ unpasteurized sauerkraut

◊ garlic (or oregano oil)

◊ 1 small piece of fresh ginger

◊ 1 lemon

◊ unpasteurized honey

◊ salt (preferably unrefined sea salt), ground coriander, ground cumin, turmeric

◊ dandelion root tincture

◊ optional: kombu seaweed, organic raw apple cider vinegar, parsley, cilantro, herbal teas (fennel, chamomile, rooibos, peppermint, holy basil, etc.)

COMING OFF THE 3 DAY CLEANSE

It is very important that you ease off The 3 Day Cleanse by gradually reintroducing healthy whole foods. Take 3 more days to work back up to a normal diet. To maintain the benefits derived from your cleanse, be sure to create new eating habits by following the recommendations in Chapter 2.

As you reintroduce foods, pay attention to how you feel. Your body may have slight or obvious reactions to foods, indicating that you might have food sensitivities. Reactions can occur within minutes or up to 48 hours later.

SELECTING A DETOXIFICATION METHOD

Each of the 3 detoxification methods described have unique benefits and will be of more use to some people than others. To choose the best method for you at this time, first determine which type(s) you are from the descriptions below and then find the appropriate detox for your type. The recommended detoxes are in order of priority from most important to least important. While combinations of types are common, there is usually a tendency toward one or two. Keep in mind that your type may change after doing one of the detoxification methods.

THE DEFICIENT TYPE

This type includes people who may be sedentary, weak, or out of shape. They have a slightly swollen, pale tongue with a thin coating, or with no coating at all. They are easily fatigued. They may be somewhat withdrawn, have low spirits, and a soft voice. Pains tend to be achy and sore.

> **Recommended Detox:** The 3 Week Cardio Detox (Note: Those with extreme deficient symptoms such as being malnourished or underweight should not do any detox. These types need to focus on tonifying and building their reserves, rather than eliminating toxins.)

THE EXCESS TYPE

This type is more outgoing and energetic. They tend to have a strong voice, and may be talkative. They may have a history of eating a lot of rich food and may be overweight. Their tongue is usually normal or red with a thick white or yellow coating. Pains tend to be more acute and extreme.

Recommended Detox: The 3 Day Cleanse, The 3 Week Cardio Detox, The 4 Week Sauna Detox.

THE HOT TYPE

This type feels warm most often and may even tend to perspire. They generally have an aversion to heat. They can be more restless. Their tongue will be red with a yellow coat, or red and dry with no coating, and may have cracks. There may also be noticeable red papillae (dots). There may be a tendency to headaches, insomnia, dizziness, high blood pressure, and anger. Complexion and eyes may be slightly red and they often have thirst. Pulse is faster.

Recommended Detox: The 3 Day Cleanse, The 3 Week Cardio Detox (The 4 Week Sauna Detox is not recommended for this type).

THE COLD TYPE

This type tends to feel chilly (preferring warmer conditions) and have a pale tongue that is moist or coated white. Digestion may be weak and immunity low. Their complexion tends to be paler and they may have low blood pressure. Personality wise they are more withdrawn with a weaker voice. They feel tired and like to sleep a lot. Fear and timidity may predominate. They often have little or no thirst. Pulse is slower.

Recommended Detox: The 3 Week Cardio Detox, The 3 Day Cleanse, The 4 Week Sauna Detox.

THE DETOXIFICATION PROCESS

All forms of detoxification challenge the body, therefore it is important that you support your body with good nutrition, adequate movement, healthy lifestyle habits, and if appropriate other therapeutic measures during the process.

As the body detoxifies it is not uncommon to experience mild symptoms such as headaches, changes in bowel movements, aches and pains, fatigue, and even emotional symptoms. These symptoms are usually short—lasting a few hours to a day—and are typically considered a normal part of "cleaning house".

One way to ensure comfort during detoxification is to go *slowly* with the process. The detoxification programs outlined in this chapter are designed to create gradual change. Follow the guidelines as described and you will ensure an effective and comfortable process.

If you experience any intense or long lasting symptoms, slow down or stop the process and resume when symptoms abate. Check in with a qualified health care practitioner if needed. Be sure to maintain your other health supportive measures.

If you currently see a natural health care practitioner such as a naturopathic doctor, homeopath, herbalist, osteopath, acupuncturist, massage therapist, or chiropractor—maintain contact for additional support while undergoing any form of detoxification.

YOUR DETOXIFICATION ACTION PLAN

1. List all the ways that you can reduce or eliminate toxins from your lifestyle and environment to reduce your body's toxic burden level. _____

_____

_____

2. Choose at least one of these environmental or personal toxic exposures that you will begin eliminating or reducing starting today. _____

_____

3. When was the last time you did some cardiovascular exercise? _____

If it has been longer than a week, choose a physical activity that you can do to increase your respiration and perspiration for at least 15 minutes. _____

Commit to doing this activity within the next 24 hours.

≈ Consider doing **The 3 Week Cardio Detox**.

4. Where can you go in your community to use either a traditional or infrared sauna? _____

If medically advised and appropriate for your type, try one out this week.

≈ Consider doing **The 4 Week Sauna Detox**.

5. If appropriate for your type, choose a date you would like to do **The 3 Day Cleanse**. _____

6. Move on to *Book 2: Mind* for the next level of health and well-being!

CONCLUSION

There are countless methods available to support you on your journey. Once you embrace personal responsibility for your health and your life, you will discover how your actions and intentions shape your world. Life then becomes an exciting adventure of unlimited possibilities to explore, filled with hidden gems of opportunity—even during challenges and in murky waters of the unknown.

Life is a playground of adventure to enrich the human experience. The journey of self-healing and self-awareness provides the freedom to explore all avenues, overcome all limitations, and evolve beyond your imagination.

Let the information in this book be a starting ground for your discovery. Continue to seek and learn useful tools that support you on your journey toward optimum health and wellness.

Honor your individuality and learn to listen to your innate wisdom. This inner voice knows what is right for you and what is not. However, it can at times be clouded over by thoughts and emotions. When that happens, get grounded and quiet—move beyond the chatter, and reconnect with this part of you. Trust it. It will always guide you toward right action.

Keep life simple—and most importantly—have fun!

ABOUT THE AUTHOR

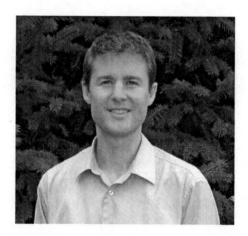

Ryan Carnahan, RMT, DCH has been practicing in the natural medicine field since 1994. He is a Registered Homeopath with a background in herbal and Chinese medicine, massage therapy, osteopathy, postural biomechanics, and energy medicine.

Ryan has always had a passionate interest in natural healing methods, and took his first course in energy medicine at age 15. He continued his studies and graduated from The Vancouver Academy of Homeopathy, The Canadian College of Massage and Hydrotherapy, and The East West School of Planetary Herbology.

Today, his intent is to share all of his knowledge about healing so others can learn to heal themselves.

Ryan has a busy practice in Port Moody, British Columbia where he works in tandem with his wife—Naturopath Dr. Kira Frketich. Visit him at www.ryancarnahan.com.

When not learning or practicing, Ryan can be found roaming the trails of the backcountry in the mountains of British Columbia, Canada.

GLOSSARY OF TERMS

CHAPTER 1

The Essentials of Health and Wellness: The most important concepts and practices required to create and maintain optimal health and wellness.

First Body Essential to Health and Wellness: Movement.

The Sedentary Lifestyle: The predominant lifestyle of modern day society consisting of very little physical movement throughout the course of a regular day. It is also the main culprit of sedentary debt and a potential contributor to health bankruptcy.

Sedentary Debt: The number of hours each day that you spend sedentary. Sedentary positions include lying or sitting down.

Health Account: Your body's bank account for health and wellness. It keeps track of your health dollars which can be deposited or withdrawn. A positive balance results in an abundance of health, vitality, longevity, and wellness. When your health account becomes depleted health bankruptcy can occur.

Health Dollars: A health credit that is capable of contributing to health and wellness. Health dollars are earned and spent by physical, mental, emotional, and spiritual actions and intentions. An abundance of health dollars keeps your health account in a positive balance.

Full Movement Potential: Your body's current and untapped capabilities for balance, strength, flexibility, endurance, and coordination.

Health Bankruptcy: A severe depletion of health dollars in your health account. Results in health problems, aches and pains, lack of energy, and a general feeling of *dis*-ease.

Postural Alignment: How your body is aligned in relation to the force of gravity. A well aligned body is balanced against gravity with all its major joints vertically and horizontally aligned. This position creates ease of movement and allows for optimal use of your full movement potential—both signs of a positive health account balance.

Regular Days: Daily movement of 15 minutes or more to pay off sedentary debt. Generally consists of easy to moderate levels of movement such as walking. Regular days do not add an abundance of health dollars to your health account, but replenish those spent during sedentary hours.

Challenge Days: Challenging types of movement performed two or more days per week for at least 15 minutes. Challenge days not only pay off sedentary debt but add an abundance of health dollars to your health account. Common types of activities performed on challenge days are running, biking, yoga, and fitness videos.

CHAPTER 2

Second Body Essential to Health and Wellness: Food.

Whole Food Diet: A diet that consists of naturally grown foods that are primarily unrefined, unprocessed, and unpackaged. The most fundamental concept of good nutrition.

The Top 6 Essentials: The 6 most important diet concepts.

Candida Albicans: A yeast that normally inhabits your intestines, but can grow out of control as a result of poor dietary habits, impaired digestion, lowered immunity, and certain medications (antibiotic, anti-inflammatory, cortisone, and birth control pills). Sugar, alcohol, and refined white flour feed Candida fungus.

Wheat Sensitivity: A food sensitivity where eating wheat causes symptoms such as mental fogginess, fatigue, skin problems (eczema, acne), and digestive symptoms such as bloating, diarrhea, and constipation. Food sensitivities are akin to minor allergies. When the sensitive food is no longer consumed—health often improves.

Cooling Foods: Foods that have a cooling effect on the body. The most common cooling foods are fruits and raw vegetables (especially bananas and melons), fruit and vegetable juices (very cooling), tofu, soy milk, bean sprouts, refrigerated foods and drinks, and frozen foods (ice cream, popsicles, ice water, etc.). Cooling foods should generally be eaten in small to moderate amounts as they can put out digestive fire.

Warming Foods: Foods that have a warming effect on the body. Warming foods include cooked foods, cooked veggies (technically still cooling but are warmer than raw), meat, fish, beans (especially black beans), whole grains, nuts and seeds, eggs, healthy oils, and butter. Warming foods, especially in the form of cooked foods, should be the bulk of most people's diet (especially in cool weather) as they assist and stoke digestive fire.

Cooling Effect: A thermal energetic principle of traditional Chinese medicine—the effect that cooling foods and other influences such as cold weather have on your physiology. Too much cold (*yin*) in the digestive system can lead to weakened digestion, gas, bloating, yeast overgrowth, aches and pains, fatigue, a tendency to feel cold, lowered immunity, and other health problems.

Warming Effect: A thermal energetic principle of traditional Chinese medicine—the effect that warming foods and other influences such as warm weather have on your physiology. Warmth (*yang*) is needed in the body for healthy digestion, good circulation, and general vitality. Too much warmth in the body (referred to as "heat") can cause headaches, high blood pressure, menopause and PMS symptoms, anger, skin eruptions, insomnia, and restlessness.

Digestive Fire: A principle of traditional Chinese medicine referring to the strength of the digestive system. A healthy digestive system has the warmth of digestive fire. Digestive fire can be put out by too many cooling foods. It can also be aggravated by too many "hot" foods such as coffee, hot spices, alcohol, and deep fried foods.

Dairy Sensitivity: A food sensitivity where eating cow dairy causes health symptoms such as digestive problems, skin problems, and fatigue. Food sensitivities are akin to minor allergies. When the sensitive food is no longer consumed—health often improves.

CHAPTER 3

Third Body Essential to Health and Wellness: Detoxification.

Homeostasis: The body's innate ability to self-regulate and heal.

Environmental Toxins: Unhealthy chemicals, substances, and influences that come from any outside source—the air you breathe, the water your drink, the food you ingest or physical contact and absorption through your skin. Unhealthy mental influences can also be classified as environmental toxins. Environmental toxins are harmful to the body/mind system and contribute to your body's toxic burden level.

Toxic Burden Level: The body's cumulative level of all the toxic substances that it is currently holding and dealing with. This includes internal toxins and those that are stored in fat cells and cell membranes. Common toxins that contribute to the body's toxic burden level include: toxic metals, pesticides, DDT, food additives, phthalates (plastics), formaldehyde, fire retardants, fumes from non-stick coatings, stain repellents, chemicals such as PCBs, and toxins released from microbes such as yeast and bacteria.

Chi: A principle of traditional Chinese medicine. Chi (or qi) is the vital life energy of the body.

Yin: A principle of traditional Chinese medicine. Yin is the cooling, nourishing, fluid aspect of the body.

Yang: A principle of traditional Chinese medicine. Yang is the warmth and strength of the body. Yang moves the circulation and warms the digestion.

Kidneys: A term used in traditional Chinese medicine that includes both the kidney organs and the adrenal glands, as well as a broad function of health and vitality. The kidneys are the house of the vital essence of health and wellness and are the root of the yin and yang in the body. They store ancestral chi and excess acquired chi.

Blood: A term used in traditional Chinese medicine that broadly includes the blood and its ability to moisten and nourish the body.

Ancestral Chi: The inherited constitutional strength of your body. According to traditional Chinese medicine, ancestral chi is stored in the kidneys. Ancestral chi can only be spent during your life—not increased.

Acquired Chi: The energy you acquire through healthy diet, proper breathing and movement, and meditative practices. An excess of acquired chi can be stored in the kidneys to prevent depletion of ancestral chi.

Sauna Therapy: The use of a sauna to stimulate detoxification of the body through perspiration and other routes of elimination. Sauna therapy can help lower the body's toxic burden level.

The 3 Step Self-Healing Protocol: A three step protocol taught in *Book 3: Spirit* that can be used for self-healing, relaxation, and Self-growth.

REFERENCES

CHAPTER 1

1. Ploughman M, 2008, Exercise is brain food: the effects of physical activity on cognitive function, *Developmental Neurorehabilitation*, Volume 11, Issue 3, pp. 236–40

2. National Center for Chronic Disease Prevention and Health Promotion, 1999, "Physical Activity and Health", *Center for Disease Control and Prevention*, http://www.cdc.gov/nccdphp/sgr/chapcon.htm (Accessed October, 2008)

3. Miyakoshi N, 2008, Daily practice using the guidelines for prevention and treatment of osteoporosis. Effectiveness of exercise for preventing and treating osteoporosis, *Clinical Calcium*, Aug;18(8), pp. 1162–8

4. Melikoglu MA, et al., 2008, The effect of regular long term training on antioxidant enzymatic activities, *The Journal of Sports Medicine and Physical Fitness*, Sep;48(3):388–90

5. Lew H, Quintanilha A, 1991, Effects of endurance training and exercise on tissue antioxidative capacity and acetaminophen detoxification, *European journal of drug metabolism and pharmacokinetics*, Jan–Mar;16(1):59–68

CHAPTER 2

1. Halweil B, 2007, "Still No Free Lunch: Nutrient levels in U.S. food supply eroded by pursuit of high yields", *The Organic Center*, http://www.organic–center.org/science.nutri.php?action=view&report_id=115 (Accessed October 2008)

2. Mayer A, 1997, Historical changes in the mineral content of fruits and vegetables, *British Food Journal*, Volume 99, Issue 6, p. 207–211(5)

Body

3. Sanchez A, et al., 1973, Role of sugars in human neutrophilic phagocytosis, *American Journal of Clinical Nutrition*, Volume 26, p:1180–1184

4. Professional Books Inc., 2003, "About Candida Yeast", *The Yeast Connection®*, http://www.yeastconnection.com/about_can_yeast.html (Accessed October 8, 2008)

5. Matsen J, 2002, *Eating Alive II*, Goodwin Books Ltd., North Vancouver, Canada, p. 496–497

6. Spinucci G, et al., 2006, Endogenous ethanol production in a patient with chronic intestinal pseudo–obstruction and small intestinal bacterial overgrowth, *European journal of gastroenterology & hepatology*, Jul;18(7):799–802

7. Professional Books Inc., 2003, "Story of The Yeast Connection", *The Yeast Connection®*, http://www.yeastconnection.com/about_story.html (Accessed October 2008)

8. Matsen J, 2002, *Eating Alive II*, Goodwin Books Ltd., North Vancouver, Canada, p. 477

9. Professional Books Inc., 2003, "Candida questionnaire and score sheet", *The Yeast Connection®*, http://www.yeastconnection.com/pdf/yeastfullsurv.pdf (Accessed October 2008)

10. Professional Books Inc., 2003, "Yeast–Fighting Program", *The Yeast Connection®*, http://www.yeastconnection.com/fighting_diet.html (Accessed October 2008)

11. Appleton N, "146 Reasons Why Sugar Is Ruining Your Health", *nancyappleton*, http://www.nancyappleton.com/NA144reasons.html (Accessed October 2008)

12. Abou–Donia MB, et al., 2008, Splenda alters gut microflora and increases intestinal p-glycoprotein and cytochrome p–450 in male rats, *Journal of toxicology and environmental health Part A*, 71(21):1415–29

13. Huff J, LaDou J, 2007, Aspartame bioassay findings portend human cancer hazards, *International Journal of Occupational and Environmental Health*, Oct–Dec;13(4):446–8

14. Reuber MD, 1978, Carcinogenicity of saccharin, *Environmental health perspectives*, August; 25: 173–200

15. Brown H, August 23, 2005, "The *Other* Brain Also Deals With Many Woes", *The New York Times*, http://www.nytimes.com/2005/08/23/health/23gut.html?pagewanted=1&_r=1 (Accessed Oct 2008)

16. Asami DK, et al., 2003, Comparison of the total phenolic and ascorbic acid content of freeze-dried and air-dried marionberry, strawberry, and corn grown using conventional, organic, and sustainable agricultural practices, *Journal of Agricultural and Food Chemistry*, Feb 26;51(5):1237–41

17. Olsson ME, et al., 2006, Antioxidant levels and inhibition of cancer cell proliferation in vitro by extracts from organically and conventionally cultivated strawberries, *Journal of Agriculture and Food Chemistry*, Feb 22;54(4):1248–55

18. Wang SY, et al., 2008, Fruit quality, antioxidant capacity, and flavonoid content of organically and conventionally grown blueberries, *Journal of Agriculture and Food Chemistry*, Jul 23;56(14):5788–94

19. Caris-Veyrat C, et al., 2004, Influence of organic versus conventional agricultural practice on the antioxidant microconstituent content of tomatoes and derived purees; consequences on antioxidant plasma status in humans, *Journal of Agriculture and Food Chemistry*, Oct 20;52(21):6503–9

20. Lu C, et al., 2008, Dietary intake and its contribution to longitudinal organophosphorus pesticide exposure in urban/suburban children, *Environmental Health Perspectives*, Apr;116(4):537–42

21. David Suzuki Foundation, 2004, "Toxins in food supply signal need for change", http://www.davidsuzuki.org/about_us/Dr_David_Suzuki/Article_Archives/weekly09030401.asp (Accessed October 2008)

22. David Suzuki Foundation, 2001, "Marine mammals face an array of ocean threats", http://www.davidsuzuki.org/About_us/Dr_David_Suzuki/Article_Archives/weekly02090101.asp (Accessed October 2008)

23. Health Canada, 2008, Food and Nutrition, "Mercury in Fish Consumption Advice: Making Informed Choices about Fish", http://www.hc-sc.gc.ca/fn-an/securit/chem-chim/environ/mercur/cons-adv-etud-eng.php (Accessed October, 2008)

24. Health Canada, 2008, Food and Nutrition, "Updating the Existing Risk Management Strategy for Mercury in Retail Fish", http://www.hc-sc.gc.ca/fn-an/pubs/mercur/risk-risque_strat-eng.php (Accessed October 2008)

25. U.S. Department of Health and Human Services and U.S. Environmental Protection Agency, May 2001 (Updated Feb 2006), "Mercury Levels in Commercial Fish and Shellfish", http://www.cfsan.fda.gov/~frf/sea-mehg.html (Accessed March 2009)

26. U.S. Food and Drug Administration, "Backgrounder for the 2004 FDA/EPA Consumer Advisory: What You Need to Know About Mercury in Fish and Shellfish", http://www.fda.gov/oc/opacom/hottopics/mercury/backgrounder.html (Accessed November 2008)

27. David Suzuki Foundation, 2004, "International farmed salmon study supports groundbreaking Suzuki Foundation research", http://www.davidsuzuki.org/Campaigns_and_Programs/Salmon_Aquaculture/News_Releases/newsaquaculture01080401.asp (Accessed Oct 2008)

28. Erasmus U, 2009, Articles, "How bad are cooking oils"?, *udoerasmus*, http://www.udoerasmus.com/articles/udo/hbaco.htm (Accessed Oct 2008)

29. Erasmus U, 1993, Fats that Heal, *Fats that Kill*, Alive Books, Burnaby, BC Canada, Page 129

30. Harvard School of Public Health, 2008, The Nutrition Source, "Shining the Spotlight on Trans Fats", http://www.hsph.harvard.edu/nutritionsource/nutrition-news/transfats/ (Accessed October 2008)

31. David Suzuki Foundation, 2003, Nature Challenge Newsletter, http://www.davidsuzuki.org/NatureChallenge/newsletters/Two.asp (Accessed October 2008)

32. Ramalho HM, et al., 2006, Effect of thermal processing on retinol levels of free-range and caged hen eggs, *International Journal of Food Sciences and Nutrition*, May–Jun;57(3–4):244–8

33. Hogervorst E, et al., 2008, High tofu intake is associated with worse memory in elderly Indonesian men and women, *Dementia and geriatric cognitive disorders*, 26(1):50–7

34. Beninger CW, Hosfield GL, 2003, Antioxidant activity of extracts, condensed tannin fractions, and pure flavonoids from Phaseolus vulgaris L. seed coat color genotypes, *Journal of Agricultural and Food Chemistry*, Dec 31;51(27):7879–83

35. Maliakal PP, Wanwimolruk S, 2001, Effect of herbal teas on hepatic drug metabolizing enzymes in rats, *The Journal of Pharmacy and Pharmacology*, Oct;53(10):1323–9

36. Lovallo WR, et al., 2005, Caffeine stimulation of cortisol secretion across the waking hours in relation to caffeine intake levels, *Psychosomatic medicine*, Sep–Oct;67(5):734–9

37. Vallejo F, et al., 2003, Phenolic compound contents in edible parts of broccoli inflorescences after domestic cooking, *Journal of the Science of Food and Agriculture*, Volume 83 Issue 14, Pages 1511–1516

38. Quan R, et al., 1992, Effects of microwave radiation on anti-infective factors in human milk, *Pediatrics*, Apr;89(4 Pt 1):667–9

39. U.S. Department of Health and Human Sciences, 2005, The Report of the Dietary Guidelines Advisory Committee on *Dietary Guidelines for Americans*, 2005, "Major Conclusions; Nutrition and your health: Dietary Guidelines for Americans", http://www.health.gov/dietaryguidelines/dga2005/report/HTML/D10_Conclusions.htm (Accessed October 2008)

CHAPTER 3

1. Health Canada, April 14 2007, Healthy Living, "The safe use of cookware, it's your health, plastics and non-stick coatings", http://www.hc-sc.gc.ca/hl-vs/iyh-vsv/prod/cook-cuisinier-eng.php (Accessed Dec 2008)

2. Crinnon WJ, 2000, Environmental medicine, part one: the human burden of environmental toxins and their common health effects, *Alternative Medicine Review: a journal of clinical therapeutic*, Feb;5(1):52–63

3. Environment News Service, 2005, "Lab Tests Find 60 Toxic Chemicals in Canadians' Blood", http://www.ens-newswire.com/ens/nov2005/2005-11-15-05.asp (Accessed Oct 2008)

4. Environmental Working Group, 2005, Body Burden - The Pollution in Newborns, "A benchmark investigation of industrial chemicals, pollutants and pesticides in umbilical cord blood", http://archive.ewg.org/reports/bodyburden2/execsumm.php (Accessed October 2008)

5. Massart F, et al., 2005, Human breast milk and xenoestrogen exposure: a possible impact on human health, *Journal of Perinatology: official journal of the California Perinatal Association*, Apr;25(4):282–8

6. Schecter A, et al., 2003, Polybrominated diphenyl ethers (PBDEs) in U.S. mothers' milk, *Environmental Health Perspectives*, Nov;111(14):1723–9

7. Lu C, et al., 2008, Dietary intake and its contribution to longitudinal organophosphorus pesticide exposure in urban/suburban children, *Environmental Health Perspectives*, Apr;116(4):537–42

8. Reyes-Herrera I, Donoghue DJ, 2008, Antibiotic residues distribute uniformly in broiler chicken breast muscle tissue, *Journal of Food Protection*, Jan;71(1):223–5

9. Villanueva CM, et al., 2004, Disinfection byproducts and bladder cancer: a pooled analysis, *Epidemiology*, May;15(3):357–67

10. Dabeka RW, et al., 2002, Survey of bottled drinking waters sold in Canada for chlorate, bromide, bromate, lead, cadmium and other trace elements, *Food additive and contaminants*, Aug;19(8):721–32

11. Kazantzis G, 2002, Mercury exposure and early effects: an overview, *La Medicina del lavoro*, May–Jun;93(3):139–47

12. Hahn LJ, et al., 1989, Dental "silver" tooth fillings: a source of mercury exposure revealed by whole-body image scan and tissue analysis, *The FASEB Journal*, 3:2641–2646

13. Health Canada, 2006, "The Safety of Dental Amalgam", http://www.hc-sc.gc.ca/dhp-mps/md-im/applic-demande/pubs/dent_amalgam-eng.php (Accessed October 2008)

14. Heavey S, June 4 2008, "Mercury teeth fillings may harm some: FDA", Reuters, http://www.reuters.com/article/healthNews/idUSN0439217520080605?feedType=RSS&feedName=healthNews&sp=true (Accessed October 2008)

15. Public Health and Agency of Canada, 2006, Table 1. Type and Contents of Vaccines Currently Approved for Use in Canada, *Canadian Immunization Guide 2006*, http://www.phac-aspc.gc.ca/publicat/cig-gci/p01-tab01-eng.php (Accessed October 2008)

16. Petrik MS, Wong MC, Tabata RC, Garry RF, Shaw CA, 2007, Aluminum adjuvant linked to Gulf War illness induces motor neuron death in mice, *Neuromolecular medicine*, 9(1):83–100

17. Generation Rescue, "About Vaccines", Chart, http://www.generationrescue.org/vaccines.html (Accessed Feb 2009)

18. Sears R, 2007, *The Vaccine Book*, Little, Brown and Company, New York, NY, USA

19. Miller D, 2004, "A User-Friendly Vaccination Schedule", *mercola*, http://articles.mercola.com/sites/articles/archive/2004/12/29/vaccination-schedule-part-one.aspx (Accessed Dec 2008)

20. Hardell L, et al., 2007, Long-term use of cellular phones and brain tumours: increased risk associated with use for ≥ 10 years, *Occupational and Environmental Medicine*, 64:626–632

21. Agarwal A, et al., 2008, Effects of radiofrequency electromagnetic waves (RF-EMW) from cellular phones on human ejaculated semen: an in vitro pilot study, *Fertility and Sterility*, Sept 18 [Epub ahead of print]

22. The City of Toronto, 2008, Healthy People Healthy Environment, "Fact Sheet - Children and Safe Cell Phone Use", http://www.toronto.ca/health/hphe/pdf/factsheet_children_safecellphone.pdf, (Accessed November 2008)

23. Divan HA, et al., 2008, Prenatal and postnatal exposure to cell phone use and behavioral problems in children, *Epidemiology (Cambridge, Mass.)*, Jul;19(4):523–9

24. Melikoglu MA, et al., 2008, The effect of regular long term training on anti-oxidant enzymatic activities, *The Journal of Sports Medicine and Physical Fitness*, Sep;48(3):388–90

25. Lew H, et al., 1991, Effects of endurance training and exercise on tissue antioxidative capacity and acetaminophen detoxification, *European journal of drug metabolism and pharmacokinetics*, Jan–Mar;16(1):59–68

26. Delarue J, et al., 2003, Fish oil prevents the adrenal activation elicited by mental stress in healthy men, *Diabetes and metabolism*, Jun;29(3):289–95

27. Schnare DW, 1986, Reduction of the human body burdens of hexachlorobenzene and polychlorinated biphenyls, *IARC scientific publications*, (77):597–603

28. Stauber JL, Florence TM, 1988, A comparative study of copper, lead, cadmium and zinc in human sweat and blood, *The Science of the Total Environment*, Aug 1;74:235–47

29. Cohn JR, Emmett EA, 1978, The excretion of trace metals in human sweat, *Annals of Clinical and Laboratory Science*, Jul–Aug;8(4):270–5

30. Sunderman FW, 1978, Clinical response to therapeutic agents in poisoning from mercury vapor, *Annals of Clinical and Laboratory Science*, Jul–Aug;8(4):259–69

31. Cirimele V, et al., 2000, Clozapine dose-concentration relationships in plasma, hair and sweat specimens of schizophrenic patients, *Forensic science international*, Jan 10;107(1–3):289–300

32. Barnes AJ, et al., 2008, Excretion of methamphetamine and amphetamine in human sweat following controlled oral methamphetamine administration, *Clinical Chemistry*, Jan;54(1):172–80

33. Zellner M, et al., 2002, Human monocyte stimulation by experimental whole body hyperthermia, *Wiener klinische Wochenschrift*, Feb 15;114(3):102-7

34. Nakano S, et al., 2007, Chlorella (Chlorella pyrenoidosa) supplementation decreases dioxin and increases immunoglobulin a concentrations in breast milk, *Journal of Medicinal Food*, Mar;10(1):134-42

35. Aga M, et al., 2001, Preventive effect of Coriandrum sativum (Chinese parsley) on localized lead deposition in ICR mice, *Journal of Ethnopharmacology*, Oct;77(2–3):203–8

36. Karunasagar D, 2005, Removal and preconcentration of inorganic and methyl mercury from aqueous media using a sorbent prepared from the plant Coriandrum sativum, *Journal of Hazardous Materials*, Feb 14;118(1–3):133–9

37. Kiruthiga PV, Shafreen RB, Pandian SK, Devi KP, 2007, Silymarin protection against major reactive oxygen species released by environmental toxins: exogenous H2O2 exposure in erythrocytes, *Basic and clinical pharmacology and toxicology*, Jun;100(6):414–9

38. Avato P, et al., 2000, Allylsulfide constituents of garlic volatile oil as antimicrobial agents, Phytomedicine: *International Journal of Phytotherapy and Phytopharmacology*, Jun;7(3):239–43

39. Weber ND, et al., 1992, In vitro virucidal effects of Allium sativum (garlic) extract and compounds, *Planta Medica*, Oct;58(5):417–23

40. Ayaz E, et al., 2008, Evaluation of the anthelmentic activity of garlic (Allium sativum) in mice naturally infected with Aspiculuris tetraptera, *Recent Patents on Anti-Infective Drug Discovery*, Jun;3(2):149–52

41. Lin HC, Pimentel M, Bacterial concepts in irritable bowel syndrome, *Reviews in gastroenterological disorders*, 2005;5 Suppl 3:S3–9

42. Tomotake H, 2006, Antibacterial Activity of Citrus Fruit Juices Against Vibrio Species, *Journal of Nutritional Science and Vitaminology*, Vol. 52, No.2 pp. 157–160

43. Gottschall E, *Food and the Gut Reaction*, The Kirkton Press, Kirkton, Ontario, Canada, pages 26–27

44. Strimpakos AS, Sharma RA, 2008, Curcumin: preventive and therapeutic properties in laboratory studies and clinical trials, *Antioxidants & redox signaling*, Mar;10(3):511–45

45. Hecht SS, 1999, Chemoprevention of cancer by isothiocyanates, modifiers of carcinogen metabolism, *The Journal of Nutrition*, Mar;129(3):768S–774S

46. Mehmetçik G, et al., 2008, Effect of pretreatment with artichoke extract on carbon tetrachloride–induced liver injury and oxidative stress, *Experimental and toxicologic pathology : official journal of the Gesellschaft für Toxikologische Pathologie*, Sep;60(6):475–80. Epub 2008 Jun 25

47. Maliakal PP, Wanwimolruk S, 2001, Effect of herbal teas on hepatic drug metabolizing enzymes in rats, *The Journal of Pharmacy and Pharmacology*, Oct;53(10):1323–9

48. Kreydiyyeh SI, Usta J, 2002, Diuretic effect and mechanism of action of parsley, *Journal of Ethnopharmacology*, Mar;79(3):353–7

INDEX